MW01118724

WATCH FOR A CLOUD OF DUST II

MORE Memories of a Dixie Veterinarian

by John E. McCormack, DVM

W.D. Hoard & Sons Company
Fort Atkinson, Wisconsin

Introduction

The title of the first volume and this book, Watch for a Cloud of Dust I & II, came about because of a former employer of Dr. McCormack, Dr. Max Foreman. An enthusiastic and excellent veterinarian, Dr. Foreman worked at a fast pace and believed in making farm calls quickly.

"Hang up the telephone and watch for a cloud of dust!" he often loudly exclaimed to a client requesting emergency service, before he sprinted to his truck and raced to the farm.

Dr. John McCormack started writing short newsletter articles on livestock health when he was a member of the Georgia Extension Service staff. His belief that all farmers and veterinarians have similar humorous experiences led to his stories in HOARD'S DAIRYMAN magazine about Carney Sam Jenkins, a bull in a wheelchair and shadetree mechanics. His first collection of stories was so popular, this second collection just had to happen.

Contents

To Jan

Whose happy smiles, positive attitude and
unwavering loyalty to her family lighten my life.
Thanks for being my wife and best friend.

1

"Is that leg broke, Doc?"

BEFORE I opened my own practice, I traveled throughout the county talking with farmers, coon dog lovers, horse enthusiasts and other potential users of veterinary service. I chatted with vo-ag teachers, the soil conservation man and spent a lot of time consulting with the county agent. Each one, without exception, either asked if I had been to see Mr. W. J. Landry or if I was going to see him. They indicated that his support of my practice would practically guarantee my success.

Mr. W. J., called Mr. "Double J" by most, owned several hundred head of purebred Herefords, a band of beautiful quarter horse mares and a kennel full of fine blue tick and redbone coon hounds. He was the owner of thousands of acres of prime southern timberland and a huge sawmill that shipped quality lumber all over the world. His elegant farm was perimetered and cross fenced with spotless white fences. When I first drove by that farm, I coveted that place!

In addition to running the farm, the sawmill and taking care of the timberland, he was chairman of the board at the bank, the savings and loan, the rural electrification organization and the county commissioners. He was a very wealthy man who also performed his civic duty with much enthusiasm. He dearly loved all his animals and, as I found out later, would spare no expense in caring for them.

When I "interviewed" him, we talked about my background, my feeling about agriculture and what I could do to help the county. He seemed to be very interested in whether or not I liked people.

"Yes," he said finally, "we do need a veterinarian in this county. If you set up here, we will use your services. As you know, we have some nice animals."

About two weeks after my official practice opening, he called late one afternoon.

"Doc, one of the boys bumped our best calf with a tractor a little while ago and hurt his front leg. He can't put any weight on it. I'd appreciate it if you could come up and take a look."

I would have preferred that my first case on his farm had been something easier. Perhaps a simple calf delivery, or a case of pinkeye or maybe even an early foot rot. I would not have selected a broken leg in a valuable bovine.

When I walked into the barn, the 300-pound Hereford calf was lying down in a large pile of straw. There were four attendants carefully monitoring his every move with concern. Mr. Landry was nervously walking, pacing back and forth and barking orders every other step.

"Careful with that leg, Eddie!" he warned. "Don't let that straw get in his eye, Fred! Watch out; don't hurt that leg! Uh, oh! He's not bloatin' up, is he, Doc? Jimmy, go get water for Doc! That leg's swole up bad, Doc! Can you give him a shot, Doc? Boy, that's the best calf we've ever raised here! Why does this always happen to the best one?"

I was already half exhausted from listening to his constant chatter, and I had not even touched the patient. When I knelt down and touched the right leg, Mr. Landry kept talking.

"Is it broke, Doc, is it broke?"

I said nothing, but just kept palpating the swollen area. When I picked up the foot with my left hand and manipulated it carefully, the calf flinched in obvious pain.

"Watch out! That hurts 'im, don't it? It's broke! I knew it!" he said, as he kept pacing and redistributing straw with his feet.

"Yessir," I said carefully, "I think it is broken. See right here just below the elbow? Feel that spot while I move this foot. You feel that grating?"

"Oh yeah, I feel it," he cried. "How bad is it, Doc?"

"Well, I can't tell for sure without an X ray, and I don't have one of . . ."

"You need an X-ray machine?" he interrupted. "We got an X-ray machine! We'll just take him down to the hospital in town and use the one down there! Let's get him loaded onto the school bus, boys!"

2

"Mr. Landry, I don't believe they'll let us X-ray a bull's leg down at the folks' hospital."

"Well, I just reckon they will!" he retorted angrily. "I bought the thing myself, I hired the administrator and I own the building. I'm also chairman of the hospital board. I believe I can X-ray anything I want to!"

Momentarily, I was stunned. I just couldn't visualize a bull being wheeled into the emergency room of the human hospital for treatment. Then I realized that he was dead serious about his authority, as well as the concern for his sick animal.

"O.K. then," I said, "why don't you go call and let them know we're coming, and we'll load the calf into the school bus."

He made a beeline to his car, a beautiful new Lincoln. But, instead of driving to the house to use the phone, he immediately produced one from between the seats. As I tranquilized the calf, I could hear his end of the conversation.

"Yes, who is this, please?" he said. "Mrs. Mosely, this is W. J. Landry. Get Walter on the phone for me, please."

We finished the injection as Mr. Landry waited quietly for Walter to get to a phone.

"Hello, Walter. W. J. here," he said authoritatively. "I've got a bull here that the vet says needs X-raying. If you don't mind we're gonna . . ."

He stopped short at that point, apparently while Walter asked a question.

"Naw, naw, a **BULL**," he emphasized. "One of my calves. He's got a broken leg!"

Again a pause while Walter responded in more detail.

"Good, I appreciate that. But no, we won't need a private room for him. We'll just get him X-rayed and perhaps use some of your stuff if Doc needs it. We'll see you in a few minutes."

In the meantime, the large crowd had commenced loading the patient through the extra large rear door of the old school bus. It was tedious work, trying to lift and push but at the same time protect the dangling leg.

"Be careful, be real careful!" ordered Mr. Landry, as he hung up the phone and sprang from the seat.

Eventually we accomplished the loading and were ready to leave. I decided to get IV fluids going before departing, so I made a venipuncture and asked one of the cowboy nurses to hold the bottle. The trip to the hospital was uneventful.

When we backed up to the emergency room door, there were several hospital employees waiting. As we opened the rear door of the bus, a young nurse came running up with a clipboard in her hand.

"What company is your insurance with?" she inquired of the cowboy. Without a moment's hesitation, he answered.

"Mr. Double J. Landry! **He's** my insurance!

2

"You can't bring that bull in this hospital"

I'LL bet there have been very few bovines brought into human hospitals for X-rays and treatment. This calf was special, however, due to its value and the unusual relationship its owner had with the hospital.

As I gazed out over my patient lying very still on the school bus floor, I could see a mass of scurrying activity at the emergency room door. There were three nurses standing nearby, one clipboarded clerical worker, an orderly and several "lookers" who just happened to drop by to observe the unusual scene after hearing about it over their CB radios.

Mr. Landry's new Lincoln, with emergency lights flashing, had preceded the slower school bus to the hospital and now was parked right up near the emergency entrance, taking up at least three prime parking spaces that normally were reserved for doctors and ambulances.

Suddenly, the emergency room door burst open, and a large rolling table being driven by two burly orderlies came barreling toward the bus. Mr. Landry was excitedly pointing and issuing orders.

"Right towards the bus, boys! Get back, people, this is an emergency! Don't crowd in, give us room! Doc, is he OK? What's his pulse? Please don't let 'im suffer! Give him another shot!"

"What insurance company was that again?" the clerk persisted.

"Look out!" cried an orderly, as he smashed into two spectators who had crowded in too close.

It was total chaos! If the patient had been a famous quarterback or a popular president, no more fuss could have been created.

By now, a police car and a deputy sheriff in a jeep had

arrived, both with blue lights flashing. The officers exited their vehicles, donned huge dark sunglasses even though it was practically night, adjusted their weapon belts and commenced crowd-control measures.

"You people back up now! Git out from under that school bus, Joe Bob! Let's make room here!" the bigger of the two lawmen ordered. The little guy ran back to his car, reached into the front seat and extracted a red bullhorn.

Flashbulbs were popping before I realized that two photographers had horned in close enough to record the soft expression on the calf's face and the irritated expression on mine. The camera operators were only representatives of the local weekly newspaper, but from their actions and the mass of equipment they had hanging from their necks, you could have erroneously deducted that they were professionals from some high-powered national magazine or news service.

"What's the animal's name? Do you suspect foul play? It has been reported that animal abuse is suspected. Do you have a comment, Doctor?" the newsmen questioned, with pens poised.

"Huh? What? Y'all talkin' to me?" I stammered. I was not used to large crowds, except at revival meetings; nor was I comfortable with picture taking and high-stress interviews.

"Yes, do you have a comment?" a reporter asked, as still another flash went off in my face.

"Yeah, I got a comment! If you flash that thing in my face one more time, I'm gonna stomp you and it both! I'm seein' spots and am half blind already!" I said, as I picked up a pair of nose tongs and faked a throw. "Just git back outa the way!"

Finally, amid much jostling and scuffling, the orderlies secured their rolling table into just the right position, and the patient was eased slowly out of the bus onto the cart. He then was covered with a large sheet.

"Hold on to this I.V., please," I requested. "Don't let that needle pull out of his vein."

More flashes popped as the patient was wheeled slowly toward the emergency room entrance. Mr. Landry was clearing a path ahead by parting the crowd with hand motions, much like Moses must have done that day when he parted the Red Sea.

When the slowly moving multitude approached the floor-operated emergency room door, it suddenly flew open, and the biggest nurse in the southeast stepped just outside and blocked our progress. She was over six feet tall, weighed about 250 pounds and had a bulldog look on her face. Her uniform was straight and stiff, no doubt from the application of at least a pound of starch.

"Why, it's Miss Juanita Peeler!" I heard someone whisper in awe. "She's the head nurse. Ain't nobody gon' mess with her!"

We all stood there, with mouths gaped open, looking up at the Amazon standing there with hands on hips. She was peering down at the crowd, looking briefly at each person, as if committing to memory each frozen face. When her gaze fell upon Mr. Landry, she started to speak.

"W. J.," she bellowed, "you know dern well that I ain't gonna let you bring no bull into my hospital."

"Juanita," Mr. W. J. stammered, "what are you doing here? I didn't know you were on duty. I thought . . ."

"Uh huh," she said, "figgered you'd slip in here, unbeknownst to me, didn't you? Well, it won't work!"

Mr. W. J. was silent. People were looking at each other, apparently afraid to speak or incur the wrath of the mammoth nurse scotched in the doorway. I decided to try my luck.

"Miss Peeler, I'm the new veterinarian in town, and we're kind of in a bind here. I don't have an X-ray machine, but we sure do need a picture of this little calf's leg. We've got him sedated so that he's not suffering right now, but when he comes around, he's gonna be in a good deal of misery. If we can't get help here in our own community, then we'll just have to drive 200 miles across the state to the veterinary school."

I noticed the two newsmen were writing frantically and shaking their heads with glee. Without really intending to, I had put her on the defensive. Now she was thinking about the stories that likely would be written about her hospital turning away a suffering patient.

"Awright," she said. Now she was talking at least four decibels lower. "Here's what we'll do. I'll have the technicians roll the mobile X-ray unit out here, and you can take the picture right here. But you can't bring that bull in this hospital!''

That was all we wanted anyway. I never really wanted to go inside the building and disrupt the tranquility of the hospital.

While we waited, I looked around at the beautiful three-story hospital. People were at nearly every window, gazing down at the goings on. I could see pajama-clad men standing with the aid of friends or crutches, looking out their windows. At other windows, I could see frail, obviously very ill elderly ladies, cranked up in their beds gazing intently, while down on the maternity wing I could see brand new mothers in beautiful pink gowns enjoying the scenery with their proud husbands. We really had created a scene.

"Doc, Doc!" Mr. Landry cried. "Let me talk with you in private for just a minute."

"I appreciate you saying what you did to Juanita," he said as we walked away from the crowd. "She and I went to school together, and we've never gotten along."

"Well, I guess we're going to get the leg X-rayed. That's what counts."

"There's something I got to ask you though, Doc," he whispered, as he looked around to be sure no one was listening. "This X-ray ain't gonna hurt reproductive function is it? I mean, you know, I've heard that X-rays will, you know what I mean, uh, cause sterility."

"Well, a couple of X-rays won't cause any problem, but just to be sure, we'll ask them to put a lead apron over his important parts," I suggested. "Then we'll be sure."

Presently, the technicians appeared, rolling out the X-ray machine. They looked at the calf warily and from every angle for at least 30 seconds before they spoke.

"What do you want done here, Doc?" they queried, as I placed the lead apron in place.

"Well, I want lateral, AP and oblique radiographs of the proximal forearm. Also, try to include the humero-radio-ulnar articulation in your view," I requested.

"Yeah, and make it snappy! We want to get him X-rayed, too!" ordered Mr. Landry.

I didn't have the nerve to tell him that an X-ray and a radiograph were the same thing!

3

"My bull in a wheelchair?"

THAT'S a strange looking radiograph," allowed a young nurse, as she sauntered into the viewing room and stared at the fresh X rays. "I've never seen a radius and ulna like that!"

"It's just a bull's leg," I said, matter-of-factly.

"A bull?" she asked, wild-eyed.

"Yeah. You know, a boy calf. A little Sunday cow!" I replied. "He's right out yonder on the emergency room patio."

She exited the room, whispering to herself and scratching her head with a pencil through a hole in her cap.

"How bad is it, Doc?" Mr. Landry queried. "Can we fix it?"

I had been studying the films with great intensity for the past several minutes. Just as I thought, both bones were broken about two inches below the elbow. The breaks were clean through, and there seemed to be no joint involvement.

A young intern had quietly eased up and also was studying the pictures. He was calculating angles with a measuring stick of some sort and was vaguely mumbling something as if quoting from some textbook on orthopedic surgery.

"What do you think should be done with that fracture, Doctor?" I asked, after he had figured for awhile.

"Well, the ulna obviously will have to be plated, of course, and . . ." He rechecked the angle of displacement, looked closely at the cortices of the bones and made several other calculations.

"Yes, the radius should be plated, also," he declared professionally. "The patient should be confined to a bed or wheelchair for at least two weeks."

"My bull in a wheelchair!" bellowed Mr. Landry. "Have you been grazin' on buckeye sprouts, young man?"

"A bu-bu-bull?" the young doctor stammered. "I thought that was the radiograph of that high school football player who was brought in here this afternoon! Aren't you his father?"

"No, I'm the vet. Do I look old enough to have a boy that old?"

Mr. Landry was on the verge of serious agitation. He had been waiting patiently at the hospital for at least an hour for a medical answer and solution to his prize calf's problem. He was not used to waiting very long for answers. I had decided what action to take, so I motioned for him to follow me outside.

"The breaks in those legs are clean, there was no splintering and there is very little over-riding," I stated. "I believe we can take him back up to the farm, make a modified Thomas splint and set that leg. You have a shop where we can fix up a splint, don't you?"

"Yes, we sure do. I'll go get the entire shop crew back in if you need 'em!" he suggested.

Two hours later, with the help of a handyman named Lee, we had fashioned a large Thomas splint out of thick aluminum rods, several pieces of flat iron and much two-inch tape and padding.

Even though the sedative was wearing off by now, we drilled four holes in the calf's outer hoof wall, threaded baling wire through the holes, attached it to the bottom of the splint and tied the ends together.

Next, we applied a dozen or so rolls of four-inch plaster of paris casting material around the leg and splint and let it dry. After we cleaned up our patient and our working area, it looked pretty nice. I felt good about the way we had the leg set and how the cast looked. My only concerns were whether or not the splint was too heavy and if the calf actually could stand and walk with the thing attached. After a little prodding, the calf sat up cow fashion and sniffed the foreign contraption that had enveloped his leg.

"He needs to sit up like this all night so he won't bloat," I suggested.

"OK, Eddie," Mr. W. J. ordered, "you stay right here and watch him until daylight. B. J., you come on in and relieve Eddie the first thing. Just be sure this calf don't lay down flat on his side. He's got to be sittin' up like this at all times. Y'all understand?''

Both young men nodded in the affirmative. They might not have understood the reason, but if Mr. Double J. issued an order, they understood that very clearly.

The next morning, I arrived at the farm about nine to find the calf standing and eating grain from a pan sitting on a folding chair. Mr. Landry was standing nearby, checking the feed to be sure it contained no foreign objects that shouldn't enter the sensitive digestive tract of his prize bull.

"Doc," he said, "the boys decided last night that this calf should be named 'Wheelchair.' Remember the doctor said that he'd need to be in a wheelchair for two weeks?"

"Wheelchair" performed quite well with his makeshift splint. He was so active and moved around so much that we kept having to add padding onto the bottom of his cast. When we finally wired on a strip of tire tread, we took care of that problem!

The photographers also paid a couple of visits to follow his progress. Eddie and B. J. both took baths, slicked up their hair with oil and put on clean overalls, so they would look nice in the picture. There were a couple of big front-page stories about "Wheelchair". The first story related the incident at the hospital and bragged on the staff for doing such a good job on the patient. Not until the very last line of the story was the patient identified as being a bovine.

A later story pictured "Wheelchair" eating alfalfa hay and looking dead at the camera, while Eddie and B. J. stood behind, grinning like possums.

Healed well . . .

When we removed the splint some six weeks later, I was afraid that healing would not be complete. However, when the saw finally removed the last piece of the filthy cast, we found that a nice callus had formed, even though the leg was a little crooked. It "toed" out just a little.

"The Lord has answered my prayers," Mr. Landry exclaimed when he saw "Wheelchair" take his first step on the leg. He still was mighty lame, but he did use that leg.

"Cocolas for everybody!" Mr. W. J. announced, " 'ceptin' you, Doc. You always drink a Dr. Pepper, don't you?"

About a year and a half later, Mr. Landry had his first production sale of breeding animals. All the animals had been shampooed and combed out. "Wheelchair" was the prettiest one there, even though I still could see a little toeing out of that front leg. However, to the casual observer, it was not apparent. Mr. Landry made an announcement when "Wheelchair" came into the sale ring.

"Y'all need to know about this fine bull," he said. "When he was just a calf, he broke his right front leg. With the help of the hospital and the best veterinarian in the county, he has healed so well that you can't tell it was ever broken."

"Wheelchair" topped the sale. I was happy since I had been called "the best vet in the county." I was on my way home several hours later when I realized that I also was the **only** vet in the county!

4

Spectacles and cows don't mix

IT'S just not fair! Large animal veterinarians shouldn't have to wear glasses. The thick, heavy ones I have to wear always are getting in my way and getting bumped and bent up when some rambunctious cow gets up in my face. Also, they are constantly being flung from their rightful resting place in front of my very near-sighted eyes.

Just this morning, I was trying to help Henry and Willie physically coerce a reluctant batch of 1,200-pound Angus cows into the alleyway behind the squeeze chute. As I whooped and hollered while standing on the side of the corral fence, I noticed an old troublemaker cow start to grin and then lunge for the fence with head lowered.

"Wham!"

The idiot cow rattled the rickety fence and the southern portion of my right leg. As I grimaced and threw my head back in moderate pain, my glasses sprang forward from the tops of my sweaty ears and landed amongst the mass of squirming bovines.

After each cow had taken her turn stomping in the general vicinity of where the glasses had gone down, they marched quietly and contently into the alleyway.

I had been nervously observing the action through squinted eyes but could see little more than large black, blurry beasts. Quickly I hopped into the pen and blindly groped around in the gummy muck for spectacle parts.

"A little to the left, Doc," suggested Willie. "Now towards you a little bit, now left."

He continued to offer directions until I finally felt something that palpated suspiciously like a temple piece and either a thick lens or the broken out bottom of a coke bottle. When I gingerly lifted the object from its undignified grave, it was covered and encased in about two pounds

13

of sticky barnyard defilement. Luckily, an old bathtub water trough was nearby so I immersed the mass in the water and commenced sloshing off the accumulated coat of crud.

After a few minutes of washing, they appeared at the top of the water like a bad picture. What a sight they were! They were covered with green, slick slime from the bottom of the water tank, and the temple pieces were pointing in opposite directions.

Luckily, the lenses weren't broken, but the left one was chipped around one edge. Crud still was adhered, like black glue, to the space between lens and frame. Further rinsing removed the slime, and then I attempted to wipe the things off on the side of my coveralls. Some careful bending with a pair of ear-tagging pliers restored them to wearable condition. When I tried them on and looked around at Willie and Henry, they both broke out in hearty guffaws!

Through a hammermill . . .

"Doc, them glasses look like they been through a hammer-mill," Henry allowed, between snickers. At least I could see now even if it was on an angle.

Actually, I hold chemistry 111 responsible for all my vision problems. When I informed my first college advisor that I wanted to become a veterinarian, he suggested that courses in chemistry would be appropriate. A couple of quarters later, he suggested that perhaps making a passing grade in chemistry 111 also would be appropriate.

My biggest problem was that I sat so far back in the lecture hall that I couldn't see the blackboard which wasn't black but green. The near-genius professor used yellow chalk which added to my poor visibility problem, as did the fact that he wrote with one hand while gleefully erasing the foggy-looking board with the other. Finally, in the spring quarter of my first year, my overburdened eyesight collapsed and I had to find optical assistance.

Since then, I have had numerous pairs of spectacles stomped, tromped, chomped, mashed, mutilated, lost in silage, baled up in hay, and a couple of pairs even deserted me while I was trying to restrain wild cows in the middle of the night.

Also, when it precipitates, they get covered with rain, snow and ice. The images I see then are all distorted and out of focus not unlike what you see in a silly mirror at the carnival.

In the wintertime, they always are fogging up because of the cold. Blood specks them up when I'm dehorning. Milk splatters on them when I'm stripping out a heifer with mastitis. But, worst of all, I simply cannot talk on the phone without having them on.

"Doc, you awake?" queried someone on the phone late the other night.

"I don't know. Let me find my specs and I'll see," I replied, as I raked knife, buckeye, keys, and various other front pocket essentials off the bedside table while palpating for the evasive glasses. Finally, I discovered them on the floor and applied them to their working position.

"Yeah, I'm awake. Whatcha need?" I answered. I really don't understand why I have to see when I'm on the telephone!

Three advantages . . .

I can think of only three advantages of wearing spectacles. First, they make you look older. This comes in handy when young vets are dealing with older farmers. They don't think 25-year-old veterinarians possibly could know very much about cows at such a tender age.

Second, wearing sunshades or glasses that change to a darker color when outside, can hide a certain amount of ignorance, as well as panic. When pondering a difficult diagnosis, or when realizing that you've just injected the incorrect antibiotic into the cow's jugular vein, the owner cannot observe the confusion, anxiety or alarm in your eyes.

Third, spectacles are called for if you require bifocals. When I went to wearing bifocals, it was a delightful experience. I could once again read my favorite magazine simply by holding it in my hand and not propped up against the wall way out in the hall. I found that I also could thread catgut into a suture needle without an assistant and read the time on my wristwatch.

Best of all though, many people tend to equate bifocals and gray hair with wisdom, the creeping experience of many, many years, and with an added amount of respect. I have noticed that, since I have been wearing these bifocals, dairymen and livestock owners are a lot better about having their cows corralled and restrained when I get to their farms. They don't often ask me to run cows down and lasso them anymore, like they did a few years ago. If I had known this, I would have gotten old sooner.

Now for those few farmers who don't ever have their stock ready when I pull up at the barn, I'm going to get a walking cane, walk bent over with lumbago and hop with toe gout when I arrive on the farm. Maybe then they'll get the message.

5

Barbershops are not just for haircuts

THIS would be a good time to get a haircut," I said to myself one afternoon as I glanced over toward the barbershop while waiting at the traffic light. I could see two waiting, while Chappell and Myatt, the two barbers, were each working over their customers' hair. Myatt saw me looking, then waved and motioned for me to come on in.

The shop was a "three-chair" affair. The first chair was not utilized except on Saturday, since most of the county folk came to town that day. Fumblin' Fred, a cotton farmer and part-time preacher from the south end of the county, cut hair at that chair. I would not allow him access to my scalp, since he shook real bad and had butchered up many a head of hair in his time. He was a poor barber but, for some reason, had a considerable following amongst his various congregations and distant relatives.

Myatt operated from the second chair, and Chappell, the owner, cut from the third. Chappell was hard of hearing, so he worked close to the radio in order to be able to hear Roy Acuff, Buck Owens and the other country music singers more clearly. The barbers were my good friends, but, the way we argued with each other, it would not have been apparent to a stranger.

As I neared the front door, I realized that I was really too dirty to be seen in a public place. I had forgotten to put on my rubber boots at the last call, so my work shoes exhibited evidence of large traces of cow manure, as did my pants and the short sleeve on the right side of my coveralls. I scraped and flicked some of the gunk off and stomped and scraped each shoe several times before opening the door.

"What you been doin', Doc?" yelled Chappell as I stepped onto the wornout linoleum on the floor.

"Aw, I had to clean off a couple of fresh cows up at Stink

Clark's place,'' I replied.

"Whatsamatter,'' growled someone in Myatt's chair. "Ain't he got no parched meal, mistletoe berry tea or turpentine?''

It was Carney Sam Jenkins! Even though he was turned in the opposite direction, I could tell from the sound of his voice that it was the county's foremost authority on foreign affairs, local political matters and homemade veterinary medicine.

Although Carney Sam's wisdom was legendary, he had difficulty understanding some of the most basic concepts of animal husbandry. He often argued with me over the need for pregnancy checking cows, establishing a controlled breeding season, the necessity for dehorning calves early in life and proper treatment for retained fetal membranes.

"I heard that Harry Moore's best bird dog died up at yo' clinic,'' said Myatt. "He have heartworms or what?''

"Naw, Harry's little girl opened the clinic front door while I was looking at the blood sample under the microscope. He ran out into the road, and the co-op feed truck hit him. When we got out there, he was graveyard dead.''

"I heard that Harry paid a thousand dollars for a new puppy,'' Myatt bulletined. "Is zat right?''

Source of news . . .

The thing I like most about the barbershop is that it always is an excellent source of all the latest news, hot gossip and even details of the vaguest of rumors. The Associated Press needs to go no further than the local barbershop to be completely informed of all affairs of the county, as well as any late-breaking stories of regional interest.

"I heard that Harry told Loren Caudle he was gonna go to Meridian and find hissef a new vet,'' chimed in Carney Sam. "Said he didn't figger he could afford to keep losin' dogs at the vet's here.''

Everybody snickered and looked my way to see what kind of response would be forthcoming.

"I'll tell you one thing, Dr. Carney Sam,'' I retorted. "At least I got a license to lose 'em. When are you gonna get yours?''

"Just 'cause you got a piece of fancy paper framed up on

the wall don't mean you know nothin' 'bout doctorin' on stock or huntin' dogs," Carney Sam argued.

"Well, I got the governor's signature on several papers that says different. At least I'm legal!"

Carney Sam was getting red-earred now and also getting restless in the chair. He did not like anyone criticizing him because he practiced veterinary medicine without a license, especially if it was by the one licensed practitioner in the county.

"Git up here, Doc," Chappell exclaimed, as he shook and popped the big apron. Hair flew everywhere. "While I'm cuttin' yo' hair, I need to consult with you about one of my cows."

"Awright," I allowed, "just be careful with those shears. Last time I was here you nearly skinned me." He didn't reply but, instead, started the clippers going up the back of my neck like he was combining soybeans.

"You remember my old cow that got choked on the hedgeapple, don't you?" he asked.

"Yeah, that's the one that's so old and has had so many calves."

"She's 16 years old now, and she's had 26 calves. Ten singles, five sets of twins and two sets of triplets! All born alive, too! She lost one calf to lightning, and two of the triplets fell in the creek and drowned."

"What a cow!" I marveled. "I reckon you keep her out on the back porch with her own personal bodyguard."

"Well, Sir, her teeth are wore plum down to the gum," he said, not answering. "She's thin, rough, nearly blind and got the rheumatism. Do you think I ought to sell her before winter?" He had stopped the clippers now and was leaning against the chair arm, waiting for my response.

Myatt had finished cutting Carney Sam's hair, and he was standing in front of the mirror adjusting his old, greasy Funk's G Hybrid cap on his head.

"If'n hit wuz me," Carney Sam drawled, "I'd put 'er to sleep, then send 'er to the toxidermist, have her head mounted and hang it up over these here mirrors."

"I wish he'd shut up about that cow," Myatt grumbled. "That's all I've heard about ever since she had them triplets."

If Chappell heard either one of them, he didn't let on like

he did. Sometimes being nearly deaf has its advantages.

"Chappell, if she belonged to me, I'd let her live her life out right there in that pasture behind the barn," I replied loudly. "If she gets down and we can't get her back up, then I'll give her a sleep shot, and you can bury her back on the hill."

He shook his head in agreement and went back to work.

"Doc, you gon' run for sheriff?" asked Myatt.

"What?"

"You gon' run for sheriff? Rumor has it that you're gonna try to beat Sheriff Clark."

"Naw!" I yelled. "You know better than that! How can I be sheriff and run a practice at the same time?"

"I heard the same thing up in the north end of the county yesterday," said Carney Sam. "Hit's all over the county. Some of 'em even said that you'd make a lot better lawman than horse doctor!"

I could feel my ears burning as Carney Sam exited the door and headed for his old doorless truck. As he looked back toward the barbershop, I saw him grinning and laughing while biting off a chaw of Brown's Mule.

I'm afraid that old-time barbershops are fading away from the modern scene almost as quickly as country stores. Just last week I walked into a fancy-looking place in the big city where I thought they cut hair.

"Do you have an appointment, Sir?" a strange-looking person asked as he sashayed up to my side. On his name tag it said "Mr. James".

"An appointment to get a haircut?" I asked in disbelief. "I didn't know I had to call ahead!"

"Perhaps I can squeeze you in since Mr. Charles' 10 o'clock styling and shampoo appointment may not be arriving as scheduled. Your hair does need styling badly, doesn't it?"

"Styling? Naw, I just want it cut so the boys at the feed store will quit callin' me 'Shag.' I reckon I'd better come back another time." I then fled the premises, and I have not called back for an appointment as of today.

Country stores and barbershops. I reckon feed stores will be next to disappear. Pretty soon the only place to argue and get properly insulted will be at the place where you trade trucks.

6

"Doc, you mind workin' in the rain?"

SOMETIMES I wish I had a rain thermostat. That way, when it gets real dry, we could just turn up the thermostat, and we'd be blessed with a nice shower. It would be even more helpful, though, if I could just turn that dial to stop the rain when I have a herd of cows to work.

"Doc, do you mind workin' in the rain?" the phone caller queried early one morning. It was Joe Kowalski, a tough, no-nonsense, hard working, **real** farmer. You never saw Joe drinking soda waters with the boys down at the feed store. When he did go to the feed store, he jogged into the back, told Albert the feed loader what he wanted and then quickly went on to some other business. His every waking moment was concerned with work, and he never took a day off for pleasure.

The only time I can recall ever seeing Joe even close to relaxing was the spring day his daughter got married. During the reception in the K of C hall, I found him sitting out on the back porch, sipping punch out of a fancy cup and picking at a small piece of wedding cake. He didn't even want to talk about the hog or fat steer market. I could tell that someone had secretly souped up his punch with some corn squeezins' or some other type attitude adjuster.

"I'll sure be glad to get home and get this infernal tie off," I croaked, while sticking my forefinger between the binding collar and my pinched flesh. "I'm chokin'!"

"Aw, Doc, just relax and enjoy yourself. We don't get much chance to do something like this. Step yonder and pour yourself a dipper full of this nice punch!"

Lots of times I try to line up herd work at get-togethers such as weddings, extension meetings, even after Sunday School and preaching. So I figured that this would be a good time to talk with Joe about some chute work. I sat

21

down beside him after getting my punch.

"Joe, don't you reckon it's about time to pen that herd down at the Coulter place and put 'em through the chute?" I asked. "Those calves need to be blacklegged, the heifers calfhood vaccinated and the bulls cut. The cows need lepto, IBR and . . ."

"Doc," he slurred, "I ain't gonna talk about or worry with no cows today. I just wanta sit here and be with my friends." With that, he put his arm around me and squeezed hard on that little sensitive spot between neck and shoulder.

As he maintained the paralyzing grip on my shoulder, he looked right into my face and grinned. His eyes were half shut, and his breath smelled like that of a cow with ketosis. I had seen that silly expression before, on dogs with lockjaw and on mules that had unexpectedly been lip-stuck when sampling a thistle plant.

Later, when I made calls to his farm, he never mentioned the fact that, for once in his life, he loosened up and dismissed farming from his mind for a few minutes.

So now he was calling and wanting me to work cattle in the rain so we wouldn't have to lose a "good" day working cattle when he could be plowing.

It had rained only six inches the previous 12 hours, and a lot more was coming down. The ditches were overflowing onto the highway, and vehicles passing in front of the clinic were dispatching sheets of the standing murky water at 45° angles back into the ditch banks. It was really a miserable day for cows and human beings but a pretty nice one for growing rice or frogs.

"Uh Joe," I hesitated, "I don't mind a little sprinkle, but I can't do a good job when it's pouring rain like this." I could hear the slow and steady roar of the rain on the roof. "You know yourself that it's not a good idea to be sticking cows with needles when their hides are covered with dirty old rainwater."

"Aw come on, Doc," Joe chided, "it's too wet to do any field work or paint any of the sheds."

"Joe, my Bang's vaccination charts will get all messy, and then the state veterinarian's office will write me a nasty letter. The Spotton will wash off, and the dehornings will get infected."

"Lucille said she'd fix dinner for you. Butterbeans, turnip greens, little half moon peach pies . . ." he softly recited.

"Actually, it's not raining nearly as hard as it was," I reckoned. "I suppose I could put an umbrella over my charts and put a good layer of pine tar over those horn wounds. Have you got 'em penned?"

"No, but it won't take long!" This is another oft-uttered phrase that vets hate to hear.

I never have figured out why folks want the vet on the farm before they pen the cattle.

While Joe penned cattle, I sharpened my pocket knife, hoof knives, and rearranged the drugs and equipment in the truck. Finally, they all were corralled, and we cut the cows out from the calves. The bawling increased in intensity, as well as in volume, as Mommas attempted frantically to locate their offspring by oral communication.

"Let me wire up this gate, Doc," Joe yelled as he sloshed through the mud, trying to locate a stray piece of baling wire. Where would a farmer be without baling wire or twine?

The rain had slowed to a drizzle, and I adjusted the huge red-and-black golf umbrella over the rear of my pickup truck that I had backed up adjacent to the headgate. In no time, cattle were coming through the chute, accompanied by the frantic shouts and urgings of all in attendance.

"This rain's not too bad, is it Doc?" Joe allowed two hours later when the last cow bolted from the chute. "Told you we could do it, didn't I?"

"Yep, we did it, but I still don't know why it had to be done today," I replied.

"Gotta plow tomorrow. Make haste now, Lucille will have dinner on the table by the time we get to the house and get washed up."

Sometime later, I was standing in Lucille's kitchen, chatting with her and chomping on one of her dill pickles while Joe washed up.

"Did Joe tell you why he wanted to work those cows today?" she whispered.

"No, what's up?" I whispered back.

"Our daughter is coming home from Atlanta with our new grandson. Joe is beside himself with excitement, but he doesn't want anyone to know. He's going to take off the whole day tomorrow just to play with the baby.''

"Well, isn't that just great. I am glad that he's taking time off," I answered.

I reckon working in the rain isn't too bad if you can be off from work and play with your grandchildren the next day. I wouldn't mind getting my Bang's charts soaked and a nasty letter from the state veterinarian for that!

7

Carney Sam has a "People Ph.D."

DOC! Telephone! They say it's an emergency!"

It was Walter, the town's "main" policeman. He had stuck his head into the city council conference room where we were holding our weekly Wednesday night meeting.

Tonight the big crisis was the town's overworked sewage system and the deteriorating condition of the oxidation pond. We were in the midst of discussing whether or not to hire a "sewer system consultant." Certainly something had to be done, and it had to be done quickly.

"Hate to disturb you, Doc," Walter allowed, "but Miss Jan told him to call you here."

"Who is it?" I asked.

"It's Carney Sam Jenkins. He's down at Thunder Hill working on a hawg, he says."

"Not again!" I exclaimed. "I've already been down there three times today. What's happening to all the stock there?"

Thunder Hill was 25 hard miles away from my office. At least half of those miles were unpaved which meant mud and deep dropoffs during rainy spells or washboard-like surfaces when dry. On at least three occasions that I could recall, I had slid off into the ditch and had to be dragged out by a passing pulpwood truck. Naturally, on this night it was raining.

"Carney Sam, what you up to, Boy?" I questioned loudly into the phone. I knew the phone service was pretty poor down that way.

"Zat 'chu Doc?" I heard him say in a far-off voice.

"Yeah, what is it?" I yelled back over the cracking line.

"Doc, I'm down heah at Junior Brown's place. He's got this heah big ole' fattenin' hawg that's down in his hin' end."

Junior Brown! Without a doubt, he was one of the wildest men in the county, maybe in the state! He always was drinking that home-made moonshine whiskey and doing crazy things. He had beaten up the game warden, had run the new Baptist preacher off his property and had even charged out on to the football field to challenge the referees one night during a big game. He refused to allow the state veterinarians to test his cows for brucellosis until they got a court order and assistance from the sheriff's office.

I had visited his farm twice, and both times had been disasters! A malnourished downer cow the first time. She died just as the last drop of my glucose dripped into her vein. It was a dead-on-arrival aged mule the second time. Each time I had been insulted, blamed for the poor beast's demise and not paid. I was not anxious to return to Junior Brown's place for a third time, pay or no pay!

"Can't get up at all, Carney?" I asked.

"Naw, Doc," he yelled, "he's jis' draggin' hissef aroun' and acting funny."

"What's he eating, and how big is he?" I questioned.

"Shawts 'n slop. Weighs about 500 pounds!"

Shorts and slop were the mainstays of the family porcine animal in that area. Shorts, or "middlins" as some call this feedstuff, were to the fattening hogs what grits were to the local people. This wheat-derived substance usually was added by the handful to table scraps and dishwater, then stirred with an old broom handle before being served up in a homemade, V-shaped, wooden trough.

Low in calcium . . .

The problem with this diet was that it was low in calcium and vitamin D. It often was complicated by the fact that the porker was confined to a small pen with a large coca-cola sign for a roof. As he grew, there was not enough available calcium to be absorbed into the bones. The result was weak bones or spontaneous fractures, usually of the spinal vertebrae or hip bones.

"Carney, he's probably low on calcium. Do you still have the bottle of Cal-Dextro #2 that I loaned you the other day?"

"Yeah, it's out in the truck."

"Why don't you inject that hog with about half that bottle and see if that helps. Put it under the skin," I advised.

"OK, Doc, we'll give it a try."

I knew that if the hog had a fractured bone in his back or pelvis, he probably wouldn't recover, but, if he was just low in calcium, it might get him back on his feet.

I returned to the council meeting, voted to retain the expensive services of the sewage consultant and promptly forgot about my free phone consultation with Carney Sam.

About a week later, I stopped at the Thunder Hill "Mall" for a quick noontime snack. The "Mall" consisted of Mr. Everett Thompson's general store and Tobe Long's chain-saw repair shop.

While I dined on Possum brand sardines drenched with Tabasco sauce, Mr. Everett updated me on all the details of the past week's local events. He reviewed the success of the deer hunters, ran down the list of the sick and afflicted and even knew why I was in the area that day.

As I was sopping up the last of the fiery sardines and sweating profusely under my eyes, Junior Brown came flying up on his old H Farmall tractor. He had it in road gear and the throttle wide open. He slid to a stop, locked the brakes, jumped from the tractor and headed into the store with kerosene can in hand.

"Gimme a gallon of coal oil, Everett," he growled.

"How 'bout it, Junior?" I allowed.

"Hey, Doc," he replied. "What you doin' down here?"

"Eating dinner right now," I answered. "I heard you had a sick hog the other night."

"Doc, I'm tellin' you!" he started. "That ole hawg was 'palized,' couldn't do nothin' but drag his rear end around the lot. Old Carney Sam came down here, took one look at him and gave him a whole bunch of shots."

"Did he get well?"

"Did he get well? Carney Sam's smart as a whip, Doc. He knew exactly what ailed that critter and knew exactly what medicine to give. He's good as new, runnin' around and frisky."

"Is that so?" I allowed.

"Yeah. Carney even went next door to call somebody about one of his cases before he treated my hawg. I believe he's the best vet I ever saw. You know, Doc, you could learn a heap just followin' him around!''

"You are right as rain, Junior, right as rain. He already has taught me plenty about practicing veterinary medicine.''

Carney Sam Jenkins taught me so much about the art of practice. Although he had only a third grade academic education, he possessed a Ph.D. in "interpersonal relations." That's modern-day jargon for "getting along with people!''

8

A veterinarian needs a good spouse

I REMEMBER thinking how tired I was and that both my arms felt like they had been put through a wringer. Also, someone was saying something into my ear.

"Honey, I hate to wake you, but it's time to get up."

It was my Jan, whispering softly into the ear that was out of the covers. She always has had the sweetest and most pleasant southern voice of anyone I know. Even though I was aching and still sleepy, I was being nicely revived back into consciousness.

"I know you are so tired and worn out, Dear, but Dave Barr called not long ago, and he thinks that several of those sale barn steers have shipping fever," she continued. "Are you awake?"

"Uh huh. Yeah. Sure, I'm awake," I mumbled.

"I've got coffee ready, some of that sausage you like, homemade biscuits and hot grits," she announced quietly.

Then she was gone. I could hear her little size six-and-a-half bedroom slippers tipping quietly down the carpeted hall and onto the vinyl floor of the kitchen. I could hear plates and saucers being extracted from the cabinet and the tinkle of silverware. As I continued my upward drift into consciousness, I could imagine her pouring hot, eye-opening coffee into my favorite cow cup, adding cream and sugar and setting it at just the right spot for me at the table. She was softly humming a happy tune as she flitted about the kitchen. How could she always be so pleasant, especially so early in the morning?

The phone rang, and she caught it on the first ring. Presently, she was carrying on a happy conversation with one of my clients.

"I know it," I heard her say. "He's just been working too hard and he's exhausted. I'm trying to let him sleep an extra few minutes this morning, since he had such a long day at the sale barn yesterday.''

She paused while the caller responded.

''All right, Buck, I'll tell him,'' she concluded. ''I'm sure he'll want to come by later this morning and treat her. Why don't you just hold her up in the sick pen?''

By then I had managed to get to a sitting position on the side of the bed and had paused to rest from the effort of getting there. As I sat there gathering strength, I thought about how lucky I was to have a wonderful wife like Jan.

Her husband and her children were her number one priority. How many times had I come home late, tired and dirty, only to find her patiently waiting up for me, always smiling and so happy to see me. She always made me feel like I was a special person.

How many times had her plans or work been interrupted in order to carry out mundane chores that helped me out of a bind? Like the times she had wrapped the babies in blankets and driven out to pick me up in the country when the truck broke down. Or the times she brought extra vaccine to a far-off farm, when we ran short. She always was hand carrying samples to the lab so that we could get more accurate results quickly. I just don't know how I would manage without her.

After I showered, I found clean towels laid out, then clean clothes in their usual places. Even the slightly green-armed tee shirts were in a separate pile from the nongreen stained ones. I still have some difficulty selecting the right undershirt early in the morning when my eyesight is at its worst.

The phone went off again. Just as before, she caught it on the first ring. As pleasantries were being exchanged, I walked into the kitchen, buttoning my shirt. As she scribbled on the daybook, I started to gulp down breakfast from a standing position. I knew that I had to get rolling, since the phone conversation appeared to be an emergency.

''Now, just sit down, John,'' she said with hand over the mouthpiece. ''You can spare five minutes!''

She always was concerned about proper consumption of a proper breakfast. It wasn't long though before I was receiving a big hug, and my vest was being adjusted. Then I was out the door and bolting down the driveway. When I looked back, I could see her waving from the kitchen window with one hand and reaching for dirty dishes with the other.

I believe that it takes a special kind of person to be the spouse of a veterinarian, especially if he or she is a large animal practitioner. That spouse should be vitally interested in the practice, its clients and in the special problems of those clients. There usually is a large volume of dirty and blood-stained pants, shirts and coveralls brought home. Kitchen floors get tracked up with goos, gunks and slops of various origins. Arrivals at meetings, parties and dinners usually are characterized by tardiness. Often veterinarians never arrive because of emergencies, or, if they do arrive, the phone rings or someone drives up with a convulsing dog.

In addition, veterinarians get banged around almost daily by their uncooperative large animal patients and frequently chomped upon by snarling lap dogs. Thus, their extremities always are "beat up" and traumatized. Jan can spot a bruise or detect slight hind leg lameness from 50 paces away, even in dim light.

"What's wrong with your leg, Hon?" she exclaimed in horror the other evening. I had just opened the back door and taken what I thought was a fairly normal step onto her freshly scrubbed kitchen floor.

"Aw, I don't think it amounts to much," I said. "It's just a little ole stomp bruise."

"OK, OK, let me see it," she ordered. "Hike up your britches leg!" I obeyed, reluctantly.

"Oh, my word!" she said, with hands over her mouth. "This leg looks awful! We've got to get this angry-looking bruise treated before gangrene sets in!"

Presently, she was scooping crushed ice into a double plastic sack, rummaging through the medicine cabinet, looking for some miracle liniment. Shortly thereafter, my sore leg was being cooled, palpated, rubbed, smeared and, in general, fretted over. There's no doubt that healing takes place much quicker due to good spouse attention. Thanks, Jan! You do so much for me, and I truly appreciate it!

9

"Aw, Doc, slow down a little!"

Don't read the mail while driving. You might run into another idiot!"

Sam Pete Smith, close family friend, amateur career counselor and famous champion barbeque chef, probably didn't utter the above truism. But he should have, and would have if he had thought about it.

One morning I was flying out Riderwood Road with the pedal to the metal, on the way to Scott's Mountain. Mr. Scott had called in a panic about a cow down with grass tetany. Traffic was light, as usual, so I was opening and reading through the mail that I had just picked up at the post office. There were checks from Stink Clark, Mr. W. J. Landry, Mule Murdock and the sale barn. Every few seconds, I'd look up and be sure the road was clear. I thought I was being real careful!

When I opened up a bill from a drug company, I must have stared at the atrocious balance a couple of seconds too long. The instant I looked up, the old Ford car's rear end was about three feet from my front bumper. There wasn't even time to say, "Aw, shoot!", but I did hit the brakes for an instant.

"Bam!"

It's always amazing how much racket two vehicles make when they suddenly collide. Not only is the initial explosion stunning, but the aftershock sounds of Dr. Pepper bottles hitting the dash, blood tubes shattering and various other veterinary items ricocheting around inside the truck cab are equally startling.

When the rattling and sounds of glass breaking finally subsided, I discovered that I was on the floorboard of the passenger side, looking back towards town.

"Nothing seems to be broken," I mumbled, as I palpated

legs, feet, arms and rib cage.

Finally, I was able to get into the seat, open the passenger side door and crawl out. The front of the truck was a mess! The right side of the hood was caved in, the grill looked like tossed salad and the right headlight had been enucleated and still was spinning out in the paved road, some 50 feet away. The right side of the bumper was pushed back into the fender which was only a centimeter or two from the right front tire.

When I looked at the auto, I observed that it had only a small scratch on the bumper. Nothing else was damaged. Only then did I realize that the driver was one of my neighbors, Sally Sis Simpson. She was holding the back of her neck, grimacing and whining something about "whiplash." I knew that her second cousin by marriage was a shyster lawyer in the big city. A chill shivered up my spine.

"Sally Sis, is that you? Are you OK?" I asked.

"John, what happened?" she replied, taking her hand away from her neck and walking normally in my direction. "I didn't realize it was you that hit me. I was just turning right here to take Mama up to see Aunt Icie."

"Well, I guess I was in too big a hurry and wasn't paying attention." I confessed. "But I didn't see your taillights or turn signal. Is your Mama all right?"

"Yeah, she's OK. Aw, none of them lights work," she allowed. "Billy Jack's been meanin' to fix 'em, but he stays in the woods huntin' nearly all day, and you know, he works the graveyard shift at the mill. Boy, is the front of this truck messed up!"

"Reckon we ought to call city hall and get Walter to come out here?" I said.

"Naw, he'll just come tearing out here with that stupid siren of his wide open and get everybody upset again."

I was trying to pull and bend some of the twisted metal and steel back into a position so that I could continue on to Scott's Mountain. The hood latch wouldn't work, so I went around to retrieve a halter from the back. Everything not secured or wedged in back there had slid forward and was in a big pile just behind the cab. I could see at least four broken gallon jugs of phenothiazine, and the pungent smell of horse wormer was stronger than usual. No doubt several gallons of Parvex-plus also had been smashed. There went the profit for that day!

"John, I'm so sorry about this," sobbed Sally Sis. "It's all my fault! I just knew something like this was gonna happen because of those taillights."

"You could have at least given a hand signal if you were gonna turn," I suggested.

"The window won't roll down on that side. Besides, I didn't know you were behind me, 'cause I don't have a rearview mirror."

"How in the world were you able to get an inspection sticker?"

"I don't have one," she whispered between sobs. "But as soon as I pass my driver's license test, I'll get all this fixed, one way or the other."

"Sally Sis, take your mother on up to Aunt Icie's and get off the road," I said, with shoulders drooped.

Some minutes later, with hood haltered down and fender bent out of the way of the tire, I was back on the road. When I approached the mountain, I decided to get a running start so I wouldn't have to shift gears until I got farther up the ridge.

However, just as I started up the slope, I caught sight of something out of the corner of my left eye. A grey object, flashing a white tail, whizzed into the road just as I jerked my foot off the accelerator. It was too late!

"Bam!"

At first I thought it was a large dog that had hit head-on into my left fender, but, when the antlers flopped lifelessly up on the hood, I knew that it was a deer.

I slowed to a stop, then backed up to where the big buck was lying on the road shoulder.

"Now I've got to clean and cut up this deer," I mumbled. "I don't have time for this!"

The fender was really smashed, but the truck still was driveable. I kicked pieces of chrome off to the side, dragged the animal into the back of the truck, then took off again. This time I drove slowly, keeping both eyes glued to the road and the right-of-way.

It wasn't long before I arrived at Mr. Scott's farm. I could see the cow stretched out, broadside, down in the pasture underneath the power line. The gate was open, so I pointed the truck toward the cow and bumped over the rough terrain.

As I neared my patient, I realized that her ears had not moved. That was not a good sign. Sure enough, when I sprang from the truck seat and checked for an eye wink reflex, I found that the poor cow had expired.

"Aw, shoot!" I yelled, "all those wrecks, and now I'm too late!"

I jumped into the truck, jammed the gear shift into reverse and gunned the engine. I had just turned the steering wheel and was about to step on the brake pedal when the predictable happened.

"Bam!"

"What in the world?" I hollered, rubbing the back of my head as I detrucked.

I had rammed the back of the truck into one of the huge poles supporting the electric lines overhead. The back bumper was bashed in on the side, much like its comrade up front.

"Doc, where you been?" Mr. Scott yelled as he trotted up. "My cow's done died! You told me on the phone you'd be here in 15 minutes! That was an hour and a half ago!"

"Well, I had a little trouble . . ."

"Doc, did you know that you backed into that light pole back there?" he asked, walking around behind the truck. "Wow! You really boogered up yo' back end!"

"Yessir, I know. I was in kind of a hurry, and . . ."

"And what happened to the front end? This truck is just about ruint! Doc, you ought not go runnin' around the county in somethin' like this. It's not good for your professional image!"

"Look! I was bustin' a gut to get out here to see about your cow, but I ran into a car, then a deer and now into this light pole."

"Aw, Doc, slow down a little. You always are rushin' here, rushin' there. One of these days you're gonna go off this mountain if you don't ease up a little!"

"I'll remember that, Mr. Scott, the next time you call me in a frenzy about one of your best cows that's in labor!"

I suspect that three smashups in one day is close to a record. Since that day I have slowed down, driven more carefully and rarely read the mail on my way to a call.

10

"Not a tonsillectomy on a dog?"

I HAD snared and removed the huge left tonsil from the fiery red throat of the little chihuahua and was examining closely the diseased thing in detail.

"How can a dog live with something that nasty in his throat?" I said to myself. "No wonder he has been in this clinic for treatment so many times."

As I continued mumbling, a blue Chevrolet pickup truck turned into the clinic driveway. The driver, one Happy DuPree, spied me through the surgery room window and drove right up to the building. Then he sat down on the horn for at least five seconds before he detrucked and stomped into the waiting room. He didn't stop there, though, like regular folks; instead he just barged on into the surgery room and made himself at home.

Happy was a dairyman, soybean grower and avid sportsman. He and his wife, Mary, had been blessed with three beautiful daughters but no sons.

When I opened up my practice, one of the first calls I made was to Happy's farm to work some calves. I found him to be plain spoken, outspoken and not turned in the least toward fancy phrases. After that first visit to his farm, I never was surprised at anything he said !

Somehow, Happy and I became great friends. I suppose that outside my family, Happy has been one of my closest friends. Since he had daughters, he sort of adopted me as the son he never had. He took me on my first deer hunt, taught me everything I know about catching fish and always arranged for me to get the best steak at agricultural get-togethers. He always was the "cook" at every livestock and farmer eatin' meetin'.

Great southern friends usually appear to be excessively hard on each other. To hear them argue, an outsider would think that they were only seconds away from a violent physical encounter. So, when Happy came clomping into the surgery, I knew that a great argument was only seconds away.

"How 'bout it, Happy; what you doin', Boy?" I asked.

"Aw, just slummin'," he said. "Thought I'd come by here and pay a little on that fool bill somebody sent me from this joint."

"Yeah, it was ridiculous," I apologized. "It was about half what it ought to have been. Workin' cows in that rotten old catchpen, gettin' my feet stomped, nearly gettin' gored by old cull cows, sorry help and . . ."

"Doc, did you know that dog layin' there's dead?" he stated, staring steadily at my patient. He hadn't heard a word of my insult.

"What's wrong with you, Happy? You ever seen a dead dog breathe?" I said, sarcastically, just as the little dog took a slow, deep breath.

"Well, he shore looked dead while ago," he replied. "What you doin' to 'im?"

"Taking out his tonsils. Look at that rotten tonsil right there in that basin."

"You're jokin'! Not a tonsillectomy on a dog! I never heard of such!"

"Oh yeah," I allowed, "we do this all the time. They come in here with the sore throat, coughing and gagging just like kids. When we get those bad tonsils out of there, they don't have any more problems."

"Charge 'em big" . . .

"I'll bet you charge 'em a big fee to do that, too, don't you?" he sneered.

"Naw, not much, just $50."

"**FIFTY DOLLARS!!!**" he screamed. "You mean to tell me that folks pay that?" He just stood there shaking his head back and forth. "You ought to be ashamed, taking folks' hard-earned money like that! You wouldn't catch me throwin' money away like that!"

"What do you suggest I do, Doctor DuPree, take a limb to 'em and run 'em off when they come in the door asking for help?" I asked, as I peered down into my patient's pharynx.

"Aw, Doc, you beat all . . ."

"Shh!! Shh!!" I ordered. "I need complete quiet while I'm doing this tedious surgery!" I carefully eased the remaining tonsil from its crypt and closed my snare around its base. Happy had seen all he wanted to see and now was at the receptionist's desk, writing a check and harassing Mrs. Lee.

"Cows and hogs out there dyin' in the country, and he's in 'nere fiddlin' with some rich woman's lap dog," he fumed.

"Get out of here, Happy," Mrs. Lee scolded. "You talk too much. That lap dog is just as important to those folks as your cows are to you!" She had been his neighbor all his life and had his number!

I heard the front door slam shut, then saw him crawl into his truck. As he hit the starter, he looked at me and shook his head in disgust. I motioned for him to get out of my sight.

A year or so later, Mrs. Lee called on the two-way radio with an unusual request.

"Dr. John, Happy just called and wants you to come by the house as soon as you can. He said it was an emergency, but he wouldn't let on about what it was."

"Okay, I'm just leaving Arthur Brewer's, so I'll whip by there on my way north."

I couldn't imagine what the problem could be at Happy's farm, but I knew if he called, he needed me, so I wasted no time in getting there.

When I wheeled into his driveway and skidded to a stop behind his truck, he came scurrying out the back door carrying something wrapped in a blanket. As he bounded my way, he would occasionally throw a worried look down into the wrinkled blanket.

Presently, he was truckside and was frantically uncovering a panting, wild-eyed, slobbering terrier dog.

"Dr. John, this is Glenda's little dog, and it's in a bad way," he said, sheepishly. "Glenda's off at 4-H camp, you know, and when I got home from the hayfield at dinner, this little old dog was on the verge of a conniption. She won't even let her puppies nurse. I just know she got into some of that rat poison out there on the porch!"

"Did you say puppies?"

"Yeah, she had four of 'em several days ago!"

Dose of own medicine . . .

"Uh huh," I said to myself. "She's got eclampsia and a little slow IV calcium will put her right as rain in a few minutes. But I'm gonna give him a dose of his own medicine first."

"I don't know, Happy," I said slowly. "This little old dog is running a high fever and is seriously ill. We really ought to do some blood work, take X rays, put her in intensive care. That is, if she means that much to you."

"Well, uh, yeah, Doc," he stammered. "Actually, it's Glenda's dog and . . ."

"Yeah, but we've got to do something fast! We can't wait long!"

"Well, how much is all that gonna run?" he asked.

"Probably about $50 — maybe more. I'll hold it down as much as I can," I allowed.

"Okay, go ahead Doc, and do whatever you have to do. Just try to save 'er. Glenda's little ole heart would be broke in two if this dog died on account of me!" Sweat was popping out on his forehead.

The shoe was on the other foot for a change! Perhaps now he would understand the feelings of other people who had great love for their pets.

"Before we do all that, let's give her a shot in the vein, just to see if it might give her a little relief," I suggested.

A couple of minutes later, I was slowly injecting the calcium into our patient's blood stream. Happy was as quiet as a mouse, but I knew his eyes were watching every move the little dog made.

"Okay, go put her back with her puppies, and then see if she'll drink some fresh water," I suggested some five minutes later.

I could hear him up on the screen porch, dropping pans, drawing water and bumping into chairs.

"Doc, looka here! She's drinkin'!" he yelled. "It looks like she's a heap better!"

"That's good," I said, stepping onto the porch. "I don't reckon she'll need all those X rays and stuff now, will she?

"Look, Happy," I continued, "I was just trying to prove a point with you. I proved that even a rough old hard-head like you has some feeling for a helpless creature — even if it's a lap dog.''

''I guess so, Doc, but don't you tell anybody that I agreed to spend that kind of money on 'er!''

11

Vets serve on PTA committees, too!

THE PTA meeting was dragging on and on. I carefully peeked a look at my watch, sighed and wondered if all the talking, arguing, planning and nit-picking would ever end. They had talked about teacher-parent conferences, students slipping off from school to sneak into the devilish pool room and even rehashed the controversial lunchroom policy of serving pinto beans instead of white beans.

They probably had discussed other topics, as well, but I had dozed through much of the meeting. Since it was Thursday, I had spent a long, hard day working at the sale barn 45 miles away and was in no mood for listening to debates about playground trivia.

I usually was spared the mental anguish and sitting torture of those Thursday night meetings, thanks to my heavy involvement with the livestock market on that day. Jan strongly encouraged me to attend these meetings to give her moral support since she always was the chairman or member of a covey of committees. Tonight, I had finished early and had slipped into the auditorium about 9 p.m.

Committees and boring PTA meetings are not favorite past-times of mine. In fact, I'd rather bale hay than attend a committee meeting. Working in tobacco and attending a committee meeting are about equal, in my opinion.

While I was half asleep, I heard the presiding officer call for a report from the fund-raising committee. Presently, Jan was on her feet, speaking eloquently in her usual convincing manner about the upcoming barbeque supper.

"The barbeque is taking shape nicely," she said sweetly. "John is going to get us two hogs from one of his clients up at Robjohn and transport them to the Rudder Hill hunting club barbeque pit. Then he will start cooking at mid-night the night before the event."

41

"What??" I screamed silently. "I don't remember her saying anything about me staying up all night and sweating over 400 pounds of smoking pork!" I was wide awake now, fighting panic and trying to figure out how to wiggle out of this latest civic responsibility.

"He will be calling on some of you for assistance," she now was saying. "Are there any questions?"

Doc's failures . . .

"I want to know something," said a voice from up front. "Are these hogs some of Doc's failures?" asked Clatis Tew, my pickup truck salesman buddy.

Everybody guffawed heartily while gouging their neighbors in the ribs. I was being stared at, so I grinned, too, even though my face was red with embarrassment.

A discussion followed regarding the condition of the gymnasium floor and the bids for the new stage curtain. Finally, the long-awaited motion for adjournment was mercifully heard, and dozens of people slowly attempted to stand upright after the marathon seat-numbing session.

I just had to get to the clinic and take care of the animals there, since I had not treated since that morning. So, I was hot-footing it up the aisle to the rear door, trying to get ahead of the stampede. Also, I was trying to avoid being collared by the chairman of the committee-forming committee. Too late though, I saw her cutting across the grain, between the seats, trying to time the interception of her helpless victim at about the third row from the back.

It was Miss Mary Belle Evans, long-time civic leader and perennial seeker of committee workers. As usual, she was carrying her old clipboard that was stuffed with papers containing the names of all her anticipated victims and their vital statistics. She had a yellow pencil stuck at an angle in a neatly done bun in the back of her blue hair and another one crossways in her mouth. The very sight of her struck terror in the hearts of all committee haters.

"All she needs is another pencil crossways through her nose," I thought to myself, "and she easily could intimidate even the meanest girl on the basketball team."

"Oh, Doctor McCormack, I must speak with you!" she ordered, "I must speak with you about an important matter at once!"

Now she had emerged from between the empty rows of seats and had her arm held straight out like a traffic cop.

I was trapped, since the exiting mass of mommas and poppas was gathering speed and bearing down on me from the rear. I surrendered and stepped to the side to await the inevitable assignment and then to begin frantic negotiations for a lesser project.

So with head bowed, lip bit and feet shuffling, I waited while Miss Mary Belle flipped through her pages of dog-eared notes.

"Ah, yes, here it is!" she allowed triumphantly. "I have you down here in charge of the program on Thursday, September 21, chairman of the legislative committee and in charge of the fund-raising deer hunt at Julian Water's hunting preserve."

As she read from the dreaded clipboard, I slowly released my lip from its toothy bite, and my mouth slowly gaped open in awe. Finally, I spoke, in a shaking and panicky voice.

"Miss Mary Belle, that's just too much! I can't do all that and work, too! You know that Thursday is my sale barn day. I can't put on a program that day!"

"Oh, of course," she apologized. "I forgot about that. Let me cross that off my agenda and make a note of that in my records for future reference."

"Yes, and also . . ."

"Oh, thank you so much for doing the very important legislative duty. I just know that you will enjoy meeting with the governor. Also, as you well know, the deer hunt raises several thousand dollars for our beloved children. You are such an asset to our community," she cooed.

"But . . ."

She quickly reached over and kissed me on the cheek. I remember that her blue hair smelled like rained-on lilacs. Then she spied another victim and quickly attacked with vigor.

"Mr. Tew, oh Mr. Clatis Tew!" she screamed softly. "I need to speak with you about an important matter!" Then she expertly sliced through the human traffic and pulled over her next sacrifice. I staggered into the cool night air, wondering what had hit me.

"Why don't they leave me alone and let me run my practice," I mumbled. "I don't have time for all this extracurricular junk!"

Four minutes later, I was inside the clinic, treating the hospitalized dogs and cats, and fuming about all the extra work that I had been assigned.

"Hey, Doc, you back there?" a loud voice suddenly shouted from the waiting room.

"Yeah, come on back!" I yelled.

It was Clatis, my good friend, and Miss Mary Belle's second victim just minutes before. As usual, he was smiling and enthusiastic.

"Good PTA meetin', wasn't it, Doc?" he asked, almost laughing. Why was he always so happy?

"Aw, Clatis, I get so tired of having to do all this extra civic work. I just want to do my job!" I said while examining the splint on a bird dog's leg. "Don't you resent having to do all this PTA and community work?"

"Doc, you ain't too bright for a man with all those degrees hanging up there on the wall! Don't you know there's a lot more to being part of a community than being the animal doctor? There's a lot more expected of you than that!"

"But I don't have time for all that!" I countered.

"You think you're the only one that's busy? Everybody's busy!" he yelled. "But you've got to find the time to be a barbeque cook, a fish fryer, a raffle ticket seller and a committee chairman. You've also got to donate for the new band uniforms, go to basketball games even when you don't want to and perhaps even run for public office."

"That's a lot to expect!"

"Doc, somebody did it for you when you were coming up. Now it's your turn. It's called paying your dues!"

Of course, he was absolutely right. It's not enough to just work and make a good living in a small community without accepting civic and school responsibilities. It's not always easy to participate, especially if it's on sale barn day!

12

Dentists and cows...a bad combination

I WAS nearly prone in the luxurious, red leather reclining chair, my mouth gaped open and my knuckles white as rice from death gripping the arm rests. They had an innocent looking green towel around my neck with a little chain that looked just right for choking a fellow in case he made a quick move to get up and flee. It felt like a child's bib, and I felt like a small child trapped in the electric chair.

Why is it that grown men have such an intense fear of dental offices? After all, modern, sophisticated dentistry isn't painful, is it? And modern dentists aren't torturing pain mongers are they? Then why was I filled with such dread? All the nice technician was doing was gently cleaning the stains and splotches off my decades-old but competent teeth.

My teeth always have been top notch. Only an alleged cavity or two in a couple of lower aggravating wisdom teeth years ago prevented me from possessing a perfect mouth. Dentists, dental hygienists, receptionists and passers-by have all marveled at the superb condition of my choppers. Some can't bring themselves to praise those pearly whites, though.

"Yeah, they may be good today," one dentist sneered, "but before long you'll have gum trouble." He was obviously chafed because I wouldn't help with his truck payments that year.

"They'll start falling out when you get to be 50," said another one. Well, they're still white, solid, pain-free and paymentless.

Harry Moore and Roy Cowan were the two dentists in Butler. Both were close friends and both owned good hunting dogs, which required my professional services from time to time. Harry was almost a professional himself at shooting quail, and this great southern hobby requires the kenneling of several well trained pointers and setters. The veterinary care of the dogs was my responsibility and no expense was spared in that effort.

Roy was a coon hunter of statewide repute. His kennel of Blue Tick and Red Bone hounds were finely tuned coon treeing implements. They were the objects of Roy's steadfast devotion, second only to his wife and children. He made sure that his dogs had the best of everything.

Both men had been raised on small farms that produced beef cattle, and both had retained their interest in livestock. One morning I sat shaking in Harry's dental chair, while he poked around in my mouth, trying to find something to drill, pull or scrape.

"How come you got such good teeth? I can't make a living like this!" he exclaimed.

"Ungh, ahh dink otsa ilk," I tried to say. It's hard to talk with your mouth pryed open and funny-looking poking devices and cold mirrors banging around in there. Why do dentists always want to ask questions at that time?

"John, I think I'm gonna buy some cows," Harry said when he finished terrorizing my teeth.

"Sounds good to me," I replied. "Where're you getting them?"

"Thought I'd pick 'em up at the sale barn."

"Uh uh, don't do that, Harry," I warned. "All you'll get is somebody's culls. I see 'em coming through there every week; old, thin, worn out, starved carcasses. Don't do anything yet; let me see if I can find you some good-quality cow and calf pairs from one of my clients up in Sumter County."

"Well O.K., but I'm ready to trade!"

I have noticed that when a man gets his mind set to trade trucks, buy cows or get married, there is no stopping him. He'll do it or bust! So when Harry called me two nights later with the news, I wasn't surprised.

"John, I got 'em!" he yelled.

"Who from?" I knew there had not been a sale that day.

"Aw, this guy over in Mississippi. Just in the edge of Lauderdale County."

"Oh no, you didn't!" I screamed. "You didn't deal with that crook down the dirt road behind the Last Chance beer garden, did you?"

"Why, yeah, that's where he lives, but . . ."

"Harry, he's got the Bang's in that herd, those cows won't milk, and they're all old as Methuselah!"

But it was too late. Harry had shelled out cash money that afternoon, and the cows were on the way, even as we spoke. He had bought not only cows, but also a passel of trouble.

The man behind the beer joint was a professional stock trader who possessed no morals, no honesty, nor any respect for livestock movement laws. Local people knew about his shyster reputation and would have nothing to do with him. However, there were enough novices and innocent first-time buyers that he continued selling diseased cows, plug horses and wormy dogs.

Just as I suspected, Harry's new herd was plagued with all sorts of problems for the next two years. I spent countless hours giving I.V. fluids to weak calves, deworming knotty yearlings and branding cows positive to the Bang's test. Finally, in frustration, Harry gave up and sold the entire herd for slaughter. It was a happy day for both of us, even though he had lost several thousand dollars.

This deal hurt him, and I am convinced that some of his gray hair sprouted because of those cows.

Not long after Harry dispersed the herd, I was in Roy's office having my teeth cleaned. As I shivered and trembled while Roy and his team of terrorists gouged and rasped on my molars, he told me the news.

"Doc, I just bought a herd of purebred Charolais cows and a bull," he announced.

"Woo hom?" I asked, from my gape-mouthed position.

"From a real nice guy over near that state line beer joint. He guaranteed 'em healthy, bred and everything!"

I slammed my mouth shut, crunching down on hard instruments and soft fingers.

"Dern, Roy, why didn't you call me before you did that? The guy's a crook! Those cows are gonna be nothing but trouble for you! Why can't I get my friends to listen to my professional advice?"

"Well, excuuuse me!" he sneered. "I didn't know I was required to check in with yo' highness before I spent my own money!"

Roy hardly spoke to me for months except at preaching every Sunday. I had just about decided that I had been wrong about that particular batch of cows. Maybe that beer joint crook had turned over a new leaf or had gotten religion. However, about nine months later, Roy called me late one night with a request.

"John, you better come down here and look at these cows. They haven't had the first calf, and I don't think they're going to!"

"No calves? I thought they were guaranteed bred!"

"Well, something's not right," he said. "I looked it up in the encyclopedia just to be sure, and it said that it takes right at nine months for a cow to have a calf."

"Have you seen the bull breed anything?"

"Not the first cow!"

I knew it! I knew something was bound to go wrong with that herd. Perhaps they were disease free but were infertile, or the bull was sterile.

Early the following Wednesday morning found us putting the big framed, fat Charolais cows through the chute. They were beautiful animals, but obviously much too fat.

The first cow was not pregnant, nor was the second, third, nor the remaining 25 head. Roy started pulling his hair out along about the sixth one, spat out his wad of Red Man on the tenth and went to the house sick on the twentieth. The worst was yet to come, however. The breeding soundness examination on the bull revealed that the 2,500-pound white wonder was sterile as a mule!

When I went to the house with the bad news, I found Roy lying down on the sofa. He was pale and shivering as he looked up at me with a pitiful look on his face.

"Uh, Roy," I said low and slow, "it's not good."

"Oh no," he groaned, "don't tell me none of the cows are pregnant!"

"I'm afraid that's correct."

"Well, why?"

"Because your bull is sterile."

"You mean that crook over there behind the beer joint . . ." he moaned.

"Yep, he sure did," I replied. "You can go see him, but I'm afraid you've been taken."

"Boy, my wife's gonna kill me. I've lost no telling how much money on those cows. All that fencin', feed, vaccine, worm medicine, association dues, fertilizer, seed, fly spray . . ."

"Well, I'm sorry, but if you had just asked me, I could have saved you all that. I know that guy real well, and he makes a living off of dentists, doctors and lawyers who want to get in the cow business."

"My accountant told me if I got some cows, I could show a loss on my income tax. Boy, was he right!"

Poor old Harry and Roy. They both lost lots of money just because they were bull-headed and thought they knew enough to match trading wits with a professional cow jockey.

Today, as my dentist checked my teeth after the hygienist had cleaned them up real good, he asked me a question.

"How's the cattle business?" he said as he removed my bib.

"Not bad," I replied, "prices are good right now."

"I've been thinking of buying several hundred cows or going into the dairy business," he said, confidently.

We talked briefly about cows, dairying and land prices. I left to make farm calls, and he went into his spotless dental chambers to crown a tooth. When I went through the waiting room, several customers were waiting.

I don't think I'll be going back to that dentist. Any dentist who is considering milking cows or raising commercial beef cattle may not be completely sane. I'm not sure I want him poking around in my mouth with those dangerous instruments.

13

Don't ever tie an animal's tail to anything

I REMEMBER it clearly. We were in a veterinary school afternoon laboratory learning about animal restraint. I was practicing a tail tie on one of the clinic animals, a middle-aged steer named Leroy.

"Don't ever tie a bull's tail to anything but himself," the tough, marine-like instructor had announced to the class.

The devilish horn flies were out in full force that September day, and they were making life miserable for both Leroy and me. He kept trying to snatch his tail away while I perfected my tail-tying technique. Occasionally, he would yank the tail out of my hands and quickly whack me in the face with the cocklebur-infested switch.

Finally, my rope and I made the perfect tail tie, and then, to celebrate my accomplishment, I looped the free end of the rope around the nearby fence post and tied it in a slipknot.

As I stood there admiring my newly acquired rope-tying skills, a horsefly the size of a hummingbird swooped down and landed right in the middle of Leroy's tenderloin. It was well known by all the class members that Leroy did not like to have his back messed with. He had kick bruised many a thigh and had raised many a painful shin splint with his lightning-like hooves in his relatively short life.

Before the giant fly even touched down good on Leroy's hide, he began fidgeting, sashaying around and tugging mightily on his tightly tied tail. It never dawned on me that a minor tragedy was imminent.

Suddenly, Leroy made a great lunge to his left, stomping the top of one daydreaming student's foot and sending another one reeling backwards into the lap of the ill-tempered professor who was demonstrating the proper method of holding up the rear foot of a cow.

Now the entire class had suspended its assignments, and each member was gazing with much interest at the disruption by the fence. At the very instant when every eye was glued to the scene, a loud ripping noise echoed throughout the barnyard. Momentarily, there was slack-jawed silence, except for the rapid wind-whistling waggings of Leroy's tail which now was a foot or so shorter than it had been only seconds earlier.

A quick glance toward the fence revealed the amputated switch still dangling, but firmly knotted, at the end of the rope. Returning my vision to poor old Leroy, I observed that blood was dripping from the stub of his tail at a rapid pace.

Immediate expulsion . . .

Finally, I slowly turned my attention toward the professor. At that moment, I assumed that I would immediately be expelled from vet school, prosecuted by the national humane society and forced to pay for a tail transplant.

The professor had come up snarling from his foot-trimming position. His face was contorted into several frowning positions as he expressed his displeasure over the tragic event.

"What idiot is responsible for this?" he barked, as he grabbed poor Leroy's tail in midswing and used his fist as a tourniquet. "Speak up! Who? Who did it?"

Chills were jumping up and down my spine like tiny racing yo-yo's, as I contemplated how I would explain my sudden arrival back home to my parents after being in school only a week or so.

Then, a strange thing happened. The professor suddenly mellowed as if touched by the magic wand of a good guy.

"It doesn't matter who did this," he said softly. "Somebody grab that bag over there, and let's get this bleeding tail stump cleaned up and wrapped."

With my heart throbbing in my throat, I darted for the black bag, handed it to him and then tried to swallow. It was difficult getting my throat muscles to work since they were constricted so tightly around my heart.

"What we'll do, troops, is apply a little of this yellow antibiotic ointment on the wound, like this," the calm professor declared. "Then place a few of these four by fours over that. Then we'll wrap it up good with this adhesive tape."

It didn't look half bad. When the tail was released, old Leroy switched it several times as if trying out a new baseball bat.

"All right, people," gently repeated the professor, "let this be a good lesson. Never tie a bull's tail to anything but himself!"

I escaped that episode without being expelled or flunking the course. I vowed that I'd never rip off a tail again!

It happened again . . .

However, 20 years later, it happened again. One of my veterinary colleagues had referred a lame Angus bull to our clinic for diagnosis and treatment. He was a high-powered, high-bred, high-strung and high-priced wonder. He had a high-class name, something like, "Black Cat of Hall Plantation." He arrived at the clinic in a fancy trailer being pulled by a large Trailways-like bus, which contained comfortable quarters for his entourage.

During the physical examination of Black Cat, I heard his value placed at $80,000; then a few minutes later, another of his attendants allowed that he was worth $125,000. When we had him safely down and securely strapped on the large operating table, the value figure went even higher.

"Somebody hang onto his tail," I asked, when he kept swishing it in my face.

The lameness problem proved to be a foot abscess which was opened quickly, drained, packed and a wooden block glued to the good claw of the affected foot. Straps were loosened, the table tilted upright and Black Cat was led away slowly. However, about the time the 2,200-pounder took his third step, I heard the same loud, ripping noise that I had heard 20 years before. Two seconds later, I felt several drops of blood as they were slung onto my face and glasses. I knew what had happened without looking.

"What idiot tied this bull's tail to the table?" I heard myself rant. "Who? Who did it?"

Silence prevailed, except for the open-mouthed gasps of the grand entourage and the swishing of the suddenly shortened tail. Also, my heart was in my throat, and I'm sure it could be heard thumping for a considerable distance.

"Well, I've done it again!" I thought to myself, "but I didn't even touch his tail this time!"

When I finally decided to peek at the "detailed" bovine, I discovered that he had ripped off only about two-thirds of the switch. There was a small tuft of short hairs left for fly-fighting purposes. I reckoned that I had to make some sort of statement to the team of attendants that encircled the patient.

"What can I say, folks?" I said slowly. "We made a mistake and tied the tail to the table."

Much to my surprise, there was no screaming and hollering; nor were knives or pistols drawn and coldly placed next to the erring veterinarian's head. Finally, the head groom spoke.

"Aw, don't worry about it, Doc," he shrugged. "What's done is done. Besides, we keep plenty of fly dope around, so he don't even need his tail anyway."

I was surprised by this remark and wondered if he were speaking on behalf of the owner. As the bus and trailer pulled out onto the highway, I had the feeling that I had not heard the last of Black Cat.

Sure enough, that night I received a phone call from the referring veterinarian.

"What happened down there today, John?" he queried. "This crowd of cowboys came by here on their way home and blessed everybody out, then went on down to the county agent's office and lit into everybody down there. What's goin' on?"

I explained to him exactly what had happened and how someone had mistakenly tied the tail to the table.

"What idiot did a stupid thing like that?" he screamed. "Didn't y'all know you were dealing with a bull worth half a million dollars?"

By some miracle, Black Cat's tail switch grew out enough that he had some abbreviated fly-fighting weaponry that summer.

Unfortunately, about two years later, Black Cat ate a four-inch piece of baling wire and died of hardware disease. Some thought he ate the wire because his tail was too short. The boys at the feed store told me that he was worth a million dollars.

That's another interesting part of dealing with animals and their owners. The value of their animals always inflates directly proportional to the severity of the injury or disease and to the degree of the veterinarian's mistake!

14

Miss Ruby's got a TV in the store!

Hello, Doctuh, are you theah?" the lady caller yelled loudly, but properly, over the phone.

"Yes, ma'am, I can hear you. Go ahead!" I replied.

"Doctuh, this is Ruby McCord," she hollered. "I need for you to stop by the stoah the next passing and examine one of my main dogs. He's gotten down in his hind end and can't get up."

"All right, Miss Ruby," I answered. "I'll stop by there tomorrow on my way back from Mr. Kent Radloff's place. Probably be about noontime."

It was Miss Ruby McCord, proprietress of "McCord's Groc. and Ser. Sta." The small country store was located between the towns of Lisman and Cromwell, and it was my favorite snack stop. Miss Ruby always had plenty of cold milk in the refrigerator, cheese on the counter, moon pies, vienna sausage, sardines and soda crackers on the shelf.

In addition to the superb, moderately priced cuisine, there were additional fringe benefits. She always kept a couple of cats inside the store, not only for companionship and her enjoyment, but for the entertainment of her guests, as well. I always purchased a little extra cheese whenever I dined there, just to be able to share it with those cats.

It was amusing, as well as relaxing, to sit reared back on a nail keg in front of the stove and toss chunks of Cheddar to the felines. To make it more challenging to them, I often would pitch the choice morsels in between two sacks of chicken feed that were propped up against the counter. All cats would dive into the crack simultaneously, each with one greedy claw extended, trying to palpate the elusive appetizer.

Another highly entertaining benefit of dining at Miss

Ruby's was the presence of human guests. It was rare to stop there and discover that no company was present. Carney Sam Jenkins, great philosopher, home-made veterinarian and gifted seer, was there frequently. Also, Buck Tutt, Cappy Lou Akins, Hoosier Turner, Bighead Turner (no relation to Hoosier) and Joe Frank Ford all were frequenters of the little oasis in the pines.

If they were all there, then most incoming customers could and should expect to be insulted, joked about, their trucks ridiculed and their hunting dogs low-rated. It was just a typical group of close southern friends. If they didn't talk badly about someone, that meant that they didn't care much for that person.

The day following Miss Ruby's phone call, I arrived at her place around 1 p.m. and discovered several vehicles there. In fact, there were so many vehicles parked around the store I wondered if something was amiss. As I de-trucked, something looked different about the place, but I couldn't put my finger on it. Suddenly, an object, bright and glowing high up over the store caught my eye. It was a TV antenna!

"Glory be! Miss Ruby's gone and put a TV in the store!" I said out loud. "Things won't ever be the same again."

Upon entering the front door, I was greeted with silence, except for the blare of the TV. Every eye was beamed right to the screen, as if hypnotized by the trashy soap opera actors hugging and kissing right there in broad daylight.

"Hey what y'all doin?" I announced.

"Hi, Doc," Joe Frank said, looking at me for a tenth of a second before quickly turning back to the screen. Not another soul uttered a word, or moved.

"Miss Ruby got a new . . ."

"Shhh, Shhh!" Carney Sam shushed me and waved me off with a frown.

Watching soaps . . .

"Now isn't this something," I mumbled, "all these tough, independent, no-nonsense, so-called farmers in here watching TV instead of home cutting off a fencerow or cleaning out the hen house."

Finally, there was a break in the action, and the dozen or

so watchers awoke from their comas, blinked their eyes and began to speak.

"What you doin' up here, Doc? Tryin' to run over some dogs?"

"Naw, he's goin' around the county sowin' blackleg seed and sprayin' the air with cholery virus."

Now, that was more like it! I felt a lot better now that the presence of the commercial had returned their sanity. Several others offered feeble attempts at insult humor.

"Doctuh, can you wait just a few minutes until this program is ovuh? This is my favorite show." Miss Ruby asked. "Then we'll go up to the house and see about Rex!"

"Whatsamatter wi' Rex, Miss Ruby?" asked Carney Sam.

"Down, can't get up. Dragging himself around."

"Uh huh, it's them kidneys! I call it kidneyitis. The kidneys drop down out of position and git chilled. It's on account of him jumpin' up on that fence and barkin' all the time." Carney Sam was beginning to roll now. He loved delivering these lectures on animal health.

"Why that's right," Miss Ruby said, stunned, "he does jump up on that fence a right smart!"

"Shh! Shh!" warned Buck. The soap was coming back on now, with another earth-shaking crisis a guaranteed feature.

Disgusted, I stood there watching the silly program with them.

"This is crazy," I thought, "watching this garbage in the middle of the afternoon while we all ought to be in the field." I couldn't stand there any longer, so I went on out to my truck and started cleaning up the drug department in the back.

A few minutes later, Miss Ruby came hopping down the steps with purse in hand, crawled into my truck, and then we were off to the house a half mile away.

"How do you like my new TV?" she asked.

"Oh, it's nice. Bet it's a lot of company for you."

"Yes, and it's one of the few coluh ones in the area. I've had a steady crowd of customuhs ever since the Sears man brought it ovuh last week."

Rex was an old Weimaraner watch dog that Miss Ruby kept in her yard. He had bedded down amongst the rose bushes near the front porch. The sickness that had struck him down in the rear end also affected his attitude since he offered no resistance when I attempted an examination.

"Is it his kidneys, Doctuh? Carney Sam said his kidneys were dropped."

"No, ma'am, I'm pretty sure it's just old age — his parts are just worn out. I'll give him a shot of old folks medicine and leave some pills. Have you given him anything?"

"I been giving him Bufferins, Bayuh aspirins, Dristan tablets and rubbing Ben-Gay on his back. Then last night I drenched him with a big dose of Hadacol."

"Why, Miss Ruby? That's not fit for a dog!"

"Well, on the television they claimed that their medicine would cure almost anything, so I decided to give it a try on old Rex here."

"You reckon it helped?" I asked.

"No, Sir, but that was befoah I knew about kidneyitis. Have you got a shot and some pills for that?"

Thank goodness for Carney Sam and color television. They both conjured up more ailments than the latest textbooks and helped me to make a good living for my family.

15

Reasons for requesting warm water

A LOT of large animal veterinarians now have nice water tanks built into their modern practice vehicles. Many even have warm water at the flick of a switch! This is all very nice and extremely convenient, but most of all, superbly professional, according to those who can afford or desire this amenity.

Actually, I have had it both ways. Some of the cars, trucks, vans and a motorcycle from which I have practiced have been unable to carry more than small quantities of water in old Army surplus cans or gallon jugs. This method often proves to be less than satisfactory since the containers frequently are empty, especially after several calls are made in rapid succession.

There are some special advantages, though, for the veterinarian to be out of water and having to ask the farmer to bring a bucket full from the creek, pond, well or house.

First, while the owner of the mysteriously ill cow, mule, pig, sheep or other domestic animal has gone to fetch the water, the puzzled veterinarian can do some quick secret reading. That's why many practitioners have some of their favorite textbooks hidden in the glove compartment, under the front seat or in one of the drug drawer compartments in the rear of the truck.

"I'll be dogged, Doc. I got a Mercury manual jus' like that one," allowed a farmer one day when he arrived back with the water sooner than expected. I was flipping quickly through the pages in my Merck manual, trying desperately to find a page, paragraph or even a phrase that matched the symptoms exhibited by the obscurely ill beast.

"Uh huh. Is that so?" I replied weakly, as I slammed the book shut, cleared my throat and quickly buried the thing deep down in my black bag.

"Just double checking on the dosage of this new medicine," I grinned. "I don't use this special medicine on anything but the best cows! This is a fine cow here! A **real** fine cow!"

However, some clients are not too pleased about the veterinarian using their barn as a place for reading. A colleague of mine was sitting on a bale of hay in a stall and frantically reading about lameness in horses one day while the owner went to get warm water. The book was so interesting that he sent the owner back to the house for a second bucket while he finished the chapter.

"Doc, I don't mind bein' your errand boy," allowed the client, "but I'll be derned if I'm gonna pay you to come out here and use my barn as a study hall! Now, do you know why this mule is lame or not?"

A second reason to send the owner to the house for warm water is so the vet can scout around in the barn and look for evidence of prior treatment. Occasionally, I have found long-necked wine bottles smeared with hog lard and reeking of turpentine hidden up amongst the rafters. An empty epsom salts box would indicate to the detective veterinarian that further use of strong purgatives would be unnecessary and probably contraindicated.

Finding a well-used O.B. sleeve wadded up and tossed into the corner might tell the practitioner that he or she wasn't the first vet to visit the case, especially if the O.B. sleeve is accompanied by a copy of a statement and an empty Banamine bottle. Adding up all this evidence will help you to better prognosticate the case or more accurately predict the outcome.

A third reason for asking for water simply is to get the client out of the barn temporarily for some reason. I remember going on a call with a certain veterinarian several years ago.

"Hurry, John, help me pull this calf," he whispered, just as the farmer exited the barn door in search of washing up water.

"Aren't we going to wait?"

"No! Hurry up! Let's deliver this calf before she has it by herself!" he argued.

In less than ten seconds, the small calf was on the ground, gasping for breath and blinking its eyes.

It wasn't long before the huffing and puffing owner bolted through the door, slinging a half bucket of water in his right hand.

"Y'all done got the calf?" he wheezed.

"Aw, yeah!" the vet replied. "Didn't look like he was gonna make it so we went ahead and delivered it. Was a tough pull, too, wasn't it, John?"

"Uh, yeah. Sure was! Uh huh!" I nodded in agreement.

"Thank goodness you were here, Doc!" the thankful farmer allowed. "She never woulda had that calf, would she?"

"Naw sir! She'd never have had that one!" the vet answered, with fingers crossed behind his back. "Good thing you called us when you did!"

The owner looked real pleased with himself, knowing that the veterinary fee had been well spent. The veterinarian looked at me and grinned a smirky half-grin, then peered cautiously upward towards the barn roof as if unsure whether or not he was going to be instantly struck down by a higher authority.

The final reason for needing fresh warm water from the house is for washing up and/or making coffee. Usually, when I ask for warm water, it is delivered to the barn smoking with steam! In that case, it is advisable to retrieve instant coffee and a cup from the black bag and enjoy a coffee break until the water turns tepid enough for washing sensitive shoulders and forearms.

Veterinarians who practice out of these up-to-date vehicles with all that modern stuff, including running water, surely do miss a lot of fun with their clients!

16

Commercials should use veterinarians

I'VE always thought that advertising agencies should hire practicing veterinarians and livestock producers to help peddle certain products. Watches, soap powders, trucks, aspirin, room fresheners and carpet cleaners are just a few of the things whose marketability could be enhanced significantly if vets and farmers would testify on behalf of those items.

The watch commercial would follow the "it took a lickin' but kept on tickin' " idea. It would be perfect with cows or hogs.

One commercial would show the cow, farmer and vet all posing proudly side by side. The farmer would be holding up a nice watch still dripping with rumen contents. He's grinning, real big like!

"Yesterday when I was feedin' up," he announces stonefaced to the camera, "this watch here fell out of the pocket of my bib overalls." Of course, he'd actually say "overhauls!"

"Fell right into the cottonseed, it did," he continues. "Old Ten Drops here run 'er tongue right out, scooped it up and swallered it like it was candy."

He fondly strokes the cow's head two or three times, while she ruminates.

"I waited for time to pass, but when it didn't, I got a hold of this veterinary here," he says, motioning toward a bespectacled green-scrub-suit clad individual standing near the rumen. It's obvious he's a large animal vet since one arm is a whole lot longer and bigger than the other. He's wiping his arms and admiring a freshly sutured incision on the side of the cow. "He rescued this watch from her innards, and it's still a runnin'!"

With that he jams the watch to his ear, listens briefly and

then holds it up for the camera to get a close-up shot so the whole world can see the second hand moving. Both men grin, and the cow softly vociferates. That's when the announcer sums it up.

"It took a chewin', but it kept on doin'!" he says.

Now, I don't know whether this will convince people to buy those watches or not, but I reckon that this ad is no worse than strapping a watch to the propeller of a motor boat and crossing the lake.

Edit detergent . . .

Soaps and detergents would be easy to sell since few people get dirtier than folks who wrestle around with stock. This commercial would open with a veterinarian's wife holding up a light-colored Sunday shirt. She can be identified as a possible veterinary wife because the gruff-looking guy standing beside her has one arm that's bigger and longer than the other.

"Honey, why do you insist on wearing your best clothes to work?" she asks, seriously. "Just look at this! There's bloodstains, cow manure, tattoo ink, mud, blue lotion, furacin ointment and bag balm all over this nice new shirt that I got down at the outlet mall! It'll never come clean!" Vet looks sheepish for a second, but recovers and makes a suggestion.

"Hey, what about this new improved 'Edit' detergent?" he exclaims, while looking at the box wistfully.

"It'll never come clean, but let's give it a try!" she sighs, dumping the grimy duds into the washer. A cupful of detergent follows the smelly clothes.

The next scene shows the smiling, long-armed vet now attired in the clean shirt that's as white as a wormy sheep's eyeballs. Mrs. Vet is palpating the shirt and is awestruck!

"Why it's a miracle!" she exclaims. "This new improved formula Edit actually got stubborn barnyard stains out of this formerly filthy shirt. Glory be!"

"It even smells fresh!" interjects the shocked husband.

"No more shirts with green-stained arms! Oh, happy day!" chirps the woman. They clinch and kiss.

The carpet-cleaning-product people are really missing a bet by not calling us in as consultants.

The commercial would show a man wearing an apron. He is pushing a vacuum cleaner over a nice white carpet when through the door stomps his veterinarian wife. Her rubber boots are covered with gunks and goos.

"Sarah! Must you track your filth into this house! Just look at my carpet! It's ruined!"

She softly backtracks to the back door, eases out of the boots and tosses them onto the back porch. Two cats slink through the cracked screen door and tromp red mud through the dining room.

Smoke appears to be streaming out of the husband's ears as he scowls and scans the scene. His once beautiful white carpet now is littered with paw and foot leavings.

Suddenly, a great hand reaches down from on high and places a small sparkling can in front of the frustrated man.

"Try new Spottoff, the miracle carpet cleaner!" booms a voice from somewhere north of the attic. "Just sprinkle on, rub in and vacuum out!"

The husband does as the voice bids. Seconds later, the once soiled carpet now is clean as a hound's tooth!

"See! Even cow lot and red clay stains virtually disappear as if by magic! Get new Spottoff today!" the big voice yells.

By this time, the couple is sitting down to the luscious supper that he has prepared. On the table can be seen pork chops, grits, greens and cathead biscuits. The cats still are inside the house but now are on the linoleum playing quietly with a toy rat. Obviously, a happy family, blessed beyond reason, because of new Spottoff.

Truck ad . . .

Pickup truck advertising is where large animal practitioners could have a great impact on sales. It is certain that if a vet's truck can withstand the abuse to which it constantly is subjected, it is worthy of their endorsement.

Commercials should show their vehicles being driven crossways over corn rows in Iowa, through knee deep Dixie mud, through door-handle-deep snow in New York and through frying sand in Arizona.

"I use this truck to chase down cows," allows a driver, obviously a veterinarian, because it says so on his door. As the uncooperative lame heifer breaks for the woods, the pickup surges forward, jumping stumps and puddles. It stops, cuts and accelerates in a manner resembling a fine cutting horse.

Finally, the heifer is turned into the barn lot, and the trusty truck comes sliding to a stop, blocking the gate. The driver jumps out, slams the door and slaps the hood a couple of times.

"If you're looking for a truck that will give you every day dependability, whether chasing bulls or negotiating swampy trails, consider this one," he says. He looks real presentable, dressed in new jeans, red vest and clean seed corn cap.

The next scene shows the same vet in the same truck, except now he's in a nice tux and has a stunning woman by his side. The truck is spotless! Even his two-way radio antenna has the crook on its end straightened out, and the bugs have been scraped off.

"See! You can take it to the annual vet convention, too!" he grins. Then he and his mate detruck and walk briskly toward the hors d' oeuvres by the pool. The camera continues to focus on the amazingly versatile truck, as other guests arrive in the background. Naturally, they all are in the same brand of trucks, and they also appear moderately to abundantly happy, even though they all have one arm that's longer than the other.

It seems to me that we do so much good advertising for those truck companies, they ought to give us free use of pickups. Perhaps I'll pursue this idea with my favorite dealership.

17

This animal died of natural causes

NO MATTER how hard livestock owners try to prevent sickness and death in their animals, they all sooner or later will suffer some death loss. We are fortunate to have good response to our vaccines when handled properly and administered to normal animals. Still, every now and then some condition pops up for which there is no prevention.

Most veterinarians strongly encourage owners to have postmortem examinations performed on those expired animals. Usually that chore is delegated to the youngest or newest associate in the practice, if it happens to be a group veterinary practice. I know that when I was a fresh graduate, it fell my lot to perform a lot of necropsies, especially on swine. Since it is not the easiest, most pleasant job that we have to perform, I would like to offer some suggestions to make it more palatable. These suggestions are for both owner and veterinarian.

1. Perform the examination as soon after death as possible. For some strange reason, most livestock deaths occur early on Saturday evening, in July, and while the owner is on a three-day, two-night trip to Florida. Most are found "up in the morning" on Monday. By then, the carcass resembles a large balloon.

"Stand back!" I barked one morning to a team of professional observers. "This thing may blow up if I make a mistake with my knife."

"Whoooosh!"

I was right! The blade had sliced into something containing a tie-splattering quantity of gas. Unfortunately for one of the watchers, his bearded face was in the direct line of fire of the accurately predicted explosion. I ducked just as the evil-odored air whistled by my ear. Incidentally, most vets develop into real good duckers. Those who don't make excellent pathologists but poor public speakers.

In a panic, the smelly faced watcher blindly groped and staggered his way towards an old trough amid the jolly shouts and yells of his cohorts, then submerged his shaking head, neck deep, into the algae-tainted water.

As usual, I was trying to stifle my giggling by keeping my head low, but I was unsuccessful. So, when he came to the surface gagging and harking, I could not help myself and surrendered to an uncontrollable attack of side-splitting guffawing.

2. Do not carry out the necropsy in the back of your new pickup or in the trunk of your spouse's car. Regardless of how careful the examination is done, a royal mess definitely will be made. It's also helpful if the deceased animal already is at its final resting place when the job is completed.

Most veterinarians I know do not ordinarily leave the carcass in exactly a cosmetically pleasing appearance. The reason for this is that once the internal body organs are extracted from their normal resting places, they seem to enlarge greatly and sometimes even multiply. There's no way they can fit back into only one carcass.

3. Necropsies should not be done out in front of the barn, in the driveway or at the neighbor's yard fenceline. Be sure you are downwind from the church, community center and schoolhouse. Dissecting a bovine alongside the interstate highway probably is not a good way to inform the general public about the finer points of veterinary medicine and livestock husbandry.

4. The veterinarian's attire is critical. No Sunday suits, golf outfits or Bermuda shorts should be worn on this job. Boots and dark coveralls are good suggestions. Also, lots of gloves should be worn since ungloved hands and arms will become green colored and smelly. Although multiple washings tend to render arms clean, spouses with extra sensitive smell systems claim that the odor penetrates the epithelial layers and even arm hair.

Amazing nose . . .

Jan can detect malodorous veterinarians from ten paces or more. She has been blessed with a gifted olfactory apparatus, and by using it she can predict exactly what I have been doing in the past 12 to 24 hours.

"Guess what I've been doing today," I stated one night as I walked in the door.

"Let's see," she said, sweetly, as she raised her nose high and sniffed several times in the air. "You posted a pig, then cleaned off a Holstein at Bud's. You ate a hot dog at the Dairy Queen sometime during the day, and you downed a least a handful of onions with it. Somewhere along the way you opened an abscess and flushed it with strong iodine solution!"

"Amazing!" I replied. "But tell me, if you are so brilliant, what kind of pig was it?"

With that she closed her eyes again and resniffed my presence.

"Smells like a crossbred gilt, probably Duroc and Piney Woods Rooter," she exclaimed.

"What a talent!"

5. It's important that proper information as to the cause of death be relayed from veterinarian to owner. Since a diagnosis frequently is not evident from the necropsy, here are a few statements that should be avoided.

"This pig died of natural causes."

Never use this line. The irate pig owner may reach for a two by four and start swinging. Vacate the premises immediately.

"His little heart just couldn't take it."

This might satisfy someone whose aged pet poodle just died from "natural causes," but it's no good on a 2,500-pound Holstein bull that destroyed fences as a hobby for years prior to his demise. Bulls just don't die of natural causes!

"Sorry, it's just too decomposed for me to tell anything."

Don't say this if you aren't sure. It could be that the poor beast had just breathed his last as you turned in at the mailbox.

"That shot I gave him yesterday didn't have anything to do with it!"

That's like waving a red flag in front of a scowling, earth-pawing bull. If the observing farmer immediately sprints toward the house and has wisps of smoke exiting from both ears, it means he has violence on his mind. Vacate the premises, pronto!

"I'm sorry, I don't have a knife."

This won't work. He'll get one from the kitchen. It probably will be even duller than the one you left behind at the last farm.

"Take these specimens of liver, lung, kidney and intestines to the house. Put them in the freezer until you can get them to the diagnostic lab."

Refrain from doing this if you want to preserve marital harmony. One time I put an entire hind leg from a deceased yearling in Jan's freezer while she was at a PTA meeting. Unfortunately, I forgot to tell her about it. The next day when she opened the door to retrieve some frozen okra, it was reported to me by one of the kids that she emitted a blood-curdling scream.

When I arrived home that night, "the leg" had created a tense atmosphere. I was informed that from then on I was prohibited from storing pathological specimens in her freezer. I neglected to tell her that the white package in the lower left corner labeled "frog legs" actually contained the brain and eyes of an old mule.

I try not to do that kind of thing any more.

18

I wanted to win the beard contest

My BEARD of eight weeks duration was giving me fits! It itched constantly and had irritated my skin beyond acceptable limits. Not only did it torment me day and night, but its appearance was hideous. Instead of matching my plain rusty red hair, it was red on the sides, brown down at my chin, white in a couple of spots on my jowls and had gray hairs liberally scattered throughout.

Everybody in town had grown beards to celebrate an upcoming bicentennial birthday of some sort. At first, I refused to quit shaving every morning, but eventually the pressure from my friends and clients became so severe that I decided to temporarily join the ranks of the unshaven.

Another problem that I encountered was that foul-smelling substances were constantly lodging within the whiskery mass. When I attended a cow that had been in labor a few hours too long, small smelly souvenirs of the extended delivery process lodged there and odored up my face until I located and washed out the culprits.

I decided that, if I were going to suffer the torment through to the final day of the celebration, I would doctor it up a little. Therefore, one night at the clinic, I took the dog clippers and a Number 40 blade and shaved my neck and the area under my chin clean. That's where sweat irritated it the most. With that done, I proceeded to clip an inch space under my nose, then cleaned up an area on each cheek. What I had then was sort of a Fu-Manchu-looking thing.

The new look was unique and was a lot better, but its stomach-turning color was still reason enough to keep me from winning the coveted prize of "best beard" on the big day. So, I decided drastic measures were in order.

Lucille Skinner ran a beauty parlor in town and also happened to be one of my favorite clients. I had seen her dogs on numerous occasions, both day and night, whenever they were sick, as well as making house calls to see her wild cats. She owed me a favor.

"Lucille, I need some help," I allowed over the phone, "but you've got to keep this quiet."

"O.K., Dr. John, what is it?"

"I need to come down there to your shop and get you to dye my beard bright red," I explained. "But I don't want Loren or Harry or anybody else to hear about it."

She agreed to keep quiet and told me to come in the back door right after noon the next day.

At the appointed hour, I parked my truck behind Sparrow's Cleaners and Laundry and, after being sure no one was watching, quietly ran across the alley, up the steps and into the back door of Skinner's Beauty Shoppe.

Even though I had never before darkened the door of a beauty parlor, I had always been curious about what the inside of one looked like. As I scanned the room, I saw several bucket-looking devices turned upside down on the backs of chairs at head level. I assumed those were hair dryers. Over to my right, I could see chairs and tables full of various hair-treating substances and several sinks. One particular sink had the appearance of a miniature dipping vat with a neck rest built into its side.

Lucille came bouncing into the room eating a Spam sandwich and drinking a Tab.

"Oh yeah, uh huh, yep, yep," she announced, thoughtfully, as she examined and palpated my beard with the expertise of a Ph.D. hairstylist. "I can see why you want something done with this wreck!"

"Can you fix it?" I asked, nervously. "I need to get out of here before somebody sees me."

"Won't take but a few minutes," she allowed. Then she pointed toward the little dipping vat. "Go yonder and sit down in that chair, put this plastic cap over your head and lay your head backwards in that basin."

Smelled like hog wormer . . .

Presently, Lucille was working some strong-smelling solution into my beard. It had the odor of shoe polish and hog wormer. As she worked it in with her fingers, she carried on a continuous commentary about the health of her pets, how brilliant they were and how much they meant to her.

Some minutes later, I was standing in front of a mirror admiring the handiwork of my personal hairdresser. The job she had done was fantastic! My beard was now the color of a Kansas City Chief football jersey — blood red!

"Perfect, Lucille!" I exclaimed. "Just what I had in mind. There's no way I can help but win the contest now!"

After some instructions from her on proper care of beards, I crept out the back door and sprinted, low to the ground, to my truck.

Many of my clients commented favorably on the condition and bright color of my beard. I was proud of it, too, now, and I was doing what I could to keep it fit for the contest on the upcoming Saturday night in the National Guard Armory. Every morning I would run my dog clippers over it very lightly in order to keep the thing even.

When the hour of the big contest finally arrived, at least 500 unshaven men were milling about on the armory floor. There were beards and goatees of all styles, sizes and colors. However, none approached mine in any way. It was undoubtedly the classiest one there.

"Our panel of female judges will select four finalists from this mob," the Chamber of Commerce man announced over the loudspeaker. "Each of you will be given a slip of paper with a number on it. If your number is called, please come to the stage." I recall that my number was 220.

As we marched around the huge room preening ourselves like strutting roosters, I could see the three judges pointing out individuals in the crowd and making various descriptive movements at their chins. After five minutes or so, a lady's voice made the announcement.

Made final four . . .

"This has been a difficult decision," she cooed, "but we have reached a consensus on the final four. Will Numbers 86, 112, 220 and 390 please report to the stage." Much applause followed, and shouts of encouragement for their favorite beard were heard from people in the audience.

When I looked around at the other three contestants, it was no contest! Not even close! They hadn't even combed theirs out or even clipped off the straggly hairs. Jack Barber's even had nasty mustard stains in the chin area! As the others were introduced, polite applause could be heard. But, when my turn came, the applause, whistling and yelling erupted into a crescendo several decibels louder than the others.

When quiet was finally restored, I noticed the town's slick-faced Baptist preacher striding swifty toward the judges' table. I smelled trouble. After a few seconds of heads-together whispering, they all looked straight at me, with lips pursed. They continued to stare, with lips now moving, and then a couple of them started to shake their heads the wrong way. I wondered what the problem could be.

"Do you reckon it has anything to do with the fact that I visited the beauty parlor?" I wondered to myself.

"Your attention, please," the pursed-lipped head judge chirped. "Your attention please! I am grieviously sorry to report that Number 220 has been disqualified from the contest."

An embarrassing hush descended upon the audience. A scattering of boos and numerous "whys" could be heard. I finally managed to speak, after the initial shock wore off.

"Why? What's the reason?" I yelled.

"It's against the rules to wear a fake beard in this event. Any beard that perfect has got to be fake!"

"This is no fake beard!" I screamed. "I've been cultivating this thing for weeks! Here, feel of it! Try to pull the hairs out!"

"No, we're not allowed to touch them," she allowed, recoiling in semihorror. "Besides, we've already decided on a winner."

"Who?" I asked, with nostrils flared. I was really steamed now.

"The winner is number 390! Mr. Jack Barber!" she smiled, leading the polite applause.

"What? What?" I bellowed to myself. "That's the one with the mustard stains all over it. There's even snuff juice stains running down from the corners of his mouth. What a revolting sight!!!"

"He's a Baptist deacon, Doc," contestant Number 86 whispered to me. "That's why the preacher came up here. He don't want us Methodists beatin' one of his prize deacons."

"Well, I'll be a suck-egg mule," I mumbled. "He's right!" The other three were all Methodists! "That preacher has quit preachin' and gone to meddlin'!!"

Within an hour, I was clipping and shaving my face clean. It was such a relief to have a cool-feeling face once again. I have shaved regularly since then and prefer it to remain that way.

Many of my friends, clients and colleagues wear beards, and they seem to be mighty proud of them. Mighty few are Methodists, though!

19

She'll be married before you know it

LISA had been seeing Mike for about a year when they announced their engagement. Naturally, we shared in their excitement and in their anticipation of a happy future life together. However, in spite of her being 24 years old, I was concerned since she still was my little girl.

It seemed just a few short years ago when she came to live with Jan and me. She was born more than a month premature, and I wasn't quite mentally prepared for her early appearance. She was so tiny, yet so beautiful, it took no time for me to be transformed into a proud, smiling, bragging father. That couldn't have been 24 years ago, could it?

Wasn't it just months ago when she would come running unsteadily through the carport when I arrived home?

"Daddee, Daddee!" she would be screaming as she leaped into my arms. Certainly any man would feel like a king with such a show of affection.

Wasn't it just weeks ago when she used to ride with me on farm calls? Sometimes she would go exploring through the barn with the farmer's children, but sometimes she stood in a feed trough, intently watching while I treated an ailing cow.

"Whatch doin', Daddy?" she would ask.

"Just giving the cow glucose."

"What's glucose?" she'd ask.

Wasn't it just a few days ago that she left for college, with her teenage enthusiasm, yet mature determination? In spite of her busy extracurricular schedule, she still found time to come home every month or so to see Daddy, Mom, the cat, and her brothers. Each time she came, she always stopped at that little roadside stand in the mountains and brought me a sack of those good boiled peanuts.

She always made sure the man triple sacked them so they'd still be hot when she arrived home. They were special for her Daddy!

Late August . . .

Both Lisa and Jan had been working for weeks on plans for the late-August wedding. There were dozens of phone calls, trips to look at dress material, trips to look at tuxedos, trips to taste samples of cake, trips to select silverware and dish designs. I never knew weddings were so chaotic, so time-consuming and so expensive! Both Jan and Lisa seemed to be in their element though, dashing here and there and discussing in detail an array of things that I thought were trivial.

"Daddy, I'll be glad when all this is over!" Lisa said late one night, after she had dragged herself into the house and collapsed on the sofa. "It's just so hectic!"

I was glad to hear someone else say out loud what I was thinking in private!

The Friday night rehearsal and dinner appeared to be going well until the bridesmaids discovered that their dresses were all wrong. Some were too long, while one was too short, and the hemline was all crooked and uneven from front to back.

Panic ensued! A frantic phone call to the dressmaker produced nothing more than a long series of unanswered rings. More panic. It was less than 18 hours until dressing time, and most of those were sleeping hours. Amid all the confusion and rapid conversation, cool-headed Jan prevailed. She decided that further telephone dialing that late in the evening not only was in poor taste, but futile as well, so the phone was given a well-deserved rest until morning.

The next morning, following a very restless night, the evasive seamstress finally was located, and arrangements were made to correct the malhemmed dresses. With garments in tow, the bridal attendants burst through all house exits and beelined toward town. The phone continued to ring at one- to two-minute intervals.

Presently, I realized that the long-standing drought had chosen that morning to come to an abrupt end. Blessed rain began plummeting to the parched earth, not in torrents, but in a semi-downpour that caused umbrellas to be retrieved in order to protect newly arranged coiffures.

Several hours later and just minutes before the ceremony, I stood tuxedoed and clean fingernailed, peering out the church fellowship hall window. I could see our friends as they drove up, parked and briskly walked through the mist into the church.

My dairy and farm family friends were almost unrecognizable since they were attired in their church-going finery, rather than coveralls, khakis, boots, and feed store caps. I could see the Daniels, the Wileys, Dan and Dorothy Cabaniss coming across the parking lot. I felt good that my clients and friends took time out at 5 p.m. to honor my family.

Suddenly, I became aware of a rustling sound and excited feminine whispering. When I turned around, I saw Lisa and her attendants entering the room, adorned in their wedding-day apparel. She was wearing the same dress that her mother had worn at our wedding nearly 30 years ago, and it was so lacey white and glistening that, when she smiled at me, she literally glowed! Jan was nervously following close behind, touching, picking and checking the dress here and there, making certain that every stitch and each shiny sequin was in its proper position. She was fretting in vain because it was flawless.

The happenings of the next few minutes are slightly blurred in my memory, but I recall hearing the organ playing the wedding march and that it made my spine tingle.

Suddenly, it was our turn and Lisa hung tightly onto my right arm as we walked slowly down the aisle. I remember thinking that there sure were a lot of people there, and they were all smiling, as they looked at us.

Soon we were standing before two robed ministers, and they were reading scriptures, making pronouncements and asking questions that required short, but serious, answers of commitment. I heard myself uttering those traditional "give away" words, and then I stepped down and joined Jan in the second row. Moments later, candles were lit, a friend read poetry, there was singing, the benediction was pronounced and the newlyweds were being applauded. All that planning and work, and now it was all over so quickly!

Some time later, after a marathon picture-taking session, we found our way to the reception hall where Lisa and Michael were cutting a four-tiered wedding cake and sampling large chunks. Multiple handshakes, hugs and messages of congratulations were being offered all over the place. It was a time and event that none of us ever will forget.

Now that it is all over, I have spent some time meditating about the role of the father of the bride. Since it is an especially difficult time for that individual, and I now have hard-earned experience in that area, I want to offer bits of advice to fathers whose beloved daughters someday likely will marry and leave home.

First, start saving for the wedding immediately! It is best to start a wedding fund before the bride's birth. In spite of exercising moderation when planning a small, but nice, wedding, the bills will still bring you to your knees. Get to know a generous banker.

Second, you will find that your friends will support you with their physical presence, and they will be concerned with your emotional health. One friend even offered to pass the hat to help with the expenses. That's a real friend!

Third, it wasn't nearly as painful as I had anticipated to put on a tuxedo, tie and other trimmings. It probably does a man good to dress up like that once in awhile.

Fourth, be sure to love and enjoy those little daughters as much as you can while you can. They will be 24 and married before you know it.

20

I was afraid they'd demand a refund

YOU ain't from aroun' hyeah, are you boy?" questioned the old man perched atop the Nehi Cola case.

"Naw, Sir, I'm not," I replied. "I missed a turn somewhere, and I'm lost. Do any of y'all know where John Tom Tew's place is?"

It was true that I probably had made wrong turns on several of the unmarked farm-to-market Alabama or Mississippi roads. I had stopped at the country store for a snack and to ask directions to a far off new farmer client who I was visiting for the first time.

I had exchanged pleasantries with the store sitters and had traded the storekeeper out of a pint of Bordens and a box of animal crackers. He claimed he didn't stock moon pies. That small amount of conversation and the fact that they didn't recognize me was enough to convince them that I was a stranger to those parts for sure.

Asking for directions is just against my principles, and so I ask only when totally confused and hopelessly uncertain as to which state or country I'm in. It's just not manly to admit to being lost and risk being considered a wimp by pleading for directions. Of course, there are exceptions, and this was one of those times.

I've found that going into a strange store and asking information as to the whereabouts of any local resident is met frequently with blank stares or profuse denials of ever hearing of anyone by that name.

"Who?" asked Sitter Number One. He squinted his eyes and looked hard in my direction. In a flat three seconds, he had examined my boots, coveralls, cap, hair color, glasses and everything else in between. I'm sure that he learned enough about me in those three seconds to present an hour seminar on my clothing sizes, health status and how many times my nose had been broken.

"John Tom Tew," I replied. "Runs a dairy around here."

"A milk dairy?" queried sitter number two. He had a confused look on his face.

Like Number One, he also sat on an upended soft drink case, but his was a Pepsi-Cola brand instead of Nehi. He was attired in "Tuf-Nut" brand overalls and had each pant leg turned up in a good 10-inch cuff. Probably bought them as long as he could get them so his wife eventually could use the extra length for patching other overalls that developed holes in their knees.

"Yes, Sir, a milk dairy," I replied, trying not to laugh or even give evidence of any humor. I've often wondered what other kind of dairy there could be, other than a "milk dairy." I suppose that's like saying "widow woman" or "tooth dentist."

"Don't nobody live 'round here by that name," said Number Two.

All heads shook in the negative, even the silent standers who weren't yet allowed a seat nor had been promoted to a position that allowed conversing with strangers. As the heads all shook from side to side, it was amusing to observe the way their eyes were riveted to my head. It was almost as if the nay saying routine was a long practiced ritual.

"Well, I don't know where I missed my turn," I allowed, looking at the crude map that John Tom had drawn for me. "He asked me to come over and consult with him about some sick cows. He's gonna be real peeved if I don't show up."

That John Tom . . .

"Oh, you mean **that** John Tom!" number one exclaimed. "Look yonder through the window. See them blue silos across the woods? That's John Tom's place."

"You some kind of cow doctor or somethin?" asked Number Two.

"Yes, Sir, I'm a veterinarian," I replied. "I don't reckon y'all have a veterinarian around here."

"Oh, yeah, we got lots of vetrans here who fool with stock in these parts," he said emphatically. "Matter of fact, Doc Kirkland lives right up the road here."

"Doctor Kirkland? I don't recall that name," I answered, somewhat perplexed at my poor memory. "Do you know where he went to vet school?"

"Well, I don't reckon he went to no school. He just taken-ed it up 'cause they was a need for it here," Number Two replied.

Presently, a debate commenced over who was the best vet in the area. Several names were mentioned, and their various strengths and weaknesses were discussed. None of the names were familiar to me. Therefore, I assumed that they were all individuals who just "took up" the practice of veterinary medicine. Finally, one of the young apprentice store sitters broke his silence and revealed his choice for best vet.

"I've heard tell of a vetnerry somewhere over yonder in Alabama," he allowed, "and he operated on some fancy bull for a rich rancher. He cut 'im open, then reached down in his innards and pulled out a six-inch piece of balin' warr with a crook on the end of it."

"Naw!" replied the shocked listeners, almost in unison.

"That's amazin'," exclaimed Number Two.

"Naw! What's amazin' is that he told 'em beforehand ex-actly what that piece of warr was gonna look like and ex-actly where it was!" said the young man, gesturing ex-citedly with his hands. "He even told 'em it'd have that crook on the end!"

"Well I know who . . . ." I said, puffing up with pride. However, I was quickly interrupted by the storekeeper. He was leaning over the counter, chewing on the stub of a cigar.

"Wonder if that was the same vet who killed Clyde Turner's cow," he queried, looking suspiciously in my direction.

I shrugged my shoulders and shook my head from side to side.

"Yeah, his ole' Jersey cow had just found a calf, and she was bad off, down and couldn't get up. He sent for this vet, and while he was givin' her a shot of calcium, her eyes walled back in her head, and she flopped over, graveyard dead."

"What'd he say?"

"He claimed it wasn't the medicine and that it was all on account of the cow had a bad heart. Said her heart was just so weak that she couldn't take it," replied the storekeeper.

"That's amazin'!" allowed one of the speakers, just as before.

"Naw! What's amazin' is that he had the gall to charge ole Clyde $30 even after he'd killed that pore old cow!"

"You know that no account vet, Mister?" asked someone.

Every head immediately turned and stared in my direction. Every eye was coldly staring daggers directly into both my eyes. There was a brief silence while I shuffled my feet.

"Uh, well, uh," I stammered, "there's several of my colleagues who work in the area. But I'm not sure who the vets are that you are referring to." I was getting nervous and beginning to sweat, so I looked at my watch, then looked up to be sure my escape route was open.

"My goodness, look at the time!" I exclaimed. "I didn't realize it was so late. John Tom will have turned all those cows out if I don't get on!"

I hit the door, waving, grinning and looking back at the unsmiling crew of sitters. It really wasn't that late, but I wanted to get out of there before I confessed to actually being the one who was responsible for the demise of Clyde Turner's cow.

I was afraid they'd gang up on me and demand a refund of that $30!

21

The pickup truck blues

THERE'S an interesting infirmity raging through the populace of this country. It appears to have originated in the southern part of the U.S. of A. among the agricultural community, but it now has spread slowly into the towns and cities even of the frigid north.

Preachers, professors and politicians are just as susceptible to this malady as farmers, football players or firemen. Although males seem to be more apt to contract it, an increasing number of females are being affected. Fortunately, it is quickly curable, although relapses every two or three years are likely. Also, the treatment becomes more expensive every year.

The condition is known as TB fever, or, in some circles, it is referred to as "The Pickup Blues." (The initials TB stand for "truck buying," not tuberculosis.) I recently suffered from a full-blown seige of it, and, although my case is in remission presently, I believe a useful purpose would be served if I informed others about this problem.

The symptoms are essentially the same, whether the victim is a first-time sufferer or a veteran of multiple attacks. Usually, the first-stage signs include depression, a feeling that one is an inferior being and an overwhelming sense of loneliness.

"Everybody's got a nice pickup but me!" the sufferer frequently is heard to utter. The statement always is spoken in anguish and frequently is accompanied by sniffling and sobbing, depending upon the present emotional level of the sufferer.

The disease then progresses into its second stage. This stage is characterized by a painful neck and jittery nerves.

The neck pain is thought to be caused by the sudden jerking and/or twisting of the head in frantic efforts to observe and covet desirable trucks as they are met on the highway. Some victims have been known to sustain severe and long-lasting cricks in their necks because of these spirited maneuvers.

Some of the nervousness comes about because of near accidents that almost occur when the victim is taking prolonged staring glances at shiney new trucks on the dealer's lot. It is quite unnerving when the sufferer returns his vision back through the windshield only to realize that his vehicle has crossed the center line. Oncoming vehicles are honking horns frantically and taking evasive action. Several episodes of this nature often will cause the harried driver to turn to strong drink, take handfuls of tranquilizers or seek solace in a dark corner of a hayloft.

The third stage is the stage of denial. The disease-ravaged individual now adamantly refuses to admit in public that he or she has TB fever.

"This truck I now have is plenty good for me," he allows, in extremely convincing tones. "It's only got 140,000 miles on it. Besides, these new trucks are just plum out of sight! It's ridiculous what they're asking for 'em!"

"We'll just get this ole' trap's transmission fixed and then paint it," he might tell his spouse. "I don't need a new one! There's no way we can afford it right now."

When the conversation contains the above-type statements or other denials of similar nature, then the astute observer should know that trading day is near.

Lowest depression . . .

The crisis nearly always comes in this third stage. This is when the depression reaches its lowest depths, and resignation to the status quo is accepted.

"Well, I don't reckon I'll ever have another nice pickup," the now seriously ill person sighs, with head down. "I'm the only one I know who doesn't have one!"

This is good because, from this point on, things gradually make a turn for the better. Sometimes, however, stage four is rough.

Stage Four is the period of shopping and shock. The initial visit to the truck dealer takes place in this stage. This first visit usually occurs late at night or on Sunday afternoon when the lot is devoid of vicious salesmen who attack the victim and stick to him like misery to poor folks.

"Oh, man, ain't this 'un pretty!" he announces, kicking at tires and softly rubbing his calloused hands over the tailgate of a red, loaded Chevy or Ford.

Seconds later, a choking, gagging sound can be heard emerging from the throat of the victim. He has just seen the price of the thing and has succumbed to "sticker shock." Some victims are staggered and knocked to their knees, as well as being struck with throat choke. Others turn and beeline it like zombies back to their old conveyances, get in and sputter off. This initial sticker shock wears off in 48 to 72 hours. They then return for further shopping, and this time they are somewhat more immune to the shock of leg-weakening high prices.

Frequently, the palms of both hands turn a dark color during this shopping period, and the tips of the forefingers become sore. This is not serious. This mysterious palm and digit affliction can be traced to a sudden interest in handling the newspaper's classified ad page and multiple dialings of the telephone.

In remission . . .

Stage Five is the period when the trade is actually made. Once this stage is reached, remission of the symptoms can practically be guaranteed. Individuals react differently during this stage. Some return to "good ole' boy" status, while others go through a mean and insulting phase, trying to squeeze out the world's best deal. They verbally attack the new truck, all its options, assail the unworthiness of the warranty and ridicule the reputation of the dealer. They make rude remarks regarding the vehicle color and complain loudly about the sound quality of the AM-FM stereo tape player entertainment center.

When a sufferer exhibits these signs, it is a sure sign that he loves the vehicle and won't draw an easy breath or sleep a sound wink until it is parked outside his bedroom window.

In Stage Six, the truck has been purchased and is in the hands of the buyer. There is absolutely no remaining sign of the disease. The depression has disappeared, and self-confidence once more has been restored.

This period is characterized by gloating, bragging and

excessive chatter. According to the now-healed victim, no one ever received a better deal on such a dynamite truck! To hear some tell it, the dealer actually paid them to take the truck.

The fuel mileage is so outstanding that the vehicle has to be stopped every few miles to let gasoline out, the air-conditioner is colder and the heater is hotter. It pulls the biggest load, never uses oil and even the entertainment center picks up that good country music station, without any static, 100 miles away over the mountain. Obviously, it wasn't assembled on a Monday since the workmanship is sober and proud.

If all goes well, there will be no flare-up of TB fever for at least two years. Some people, however, are more vulnerable and may show a relapse sooner. Others may go years without any further episodes.

Hopefully, this will serve to enlighten some of my friends who have experienced this problem but didn't know what it was. I, too, have suffered several times from this malady and have accepted the fact that I will again contract it. However, it will be a while since I just last week traded for a new white, top-of-the-line, short-bed pickup. It is loaded with every option and has the softest red seats you've ever seen!

I don't want to brag, but I just cannot believe what a deal I got on this truck! And this radio! I can pick up stations I've never heard before! The best part, though, is that I'm healthier than I've been in two years!

Since buying a truck will cure TB fever, I wonder why Blue Cross-Blue Shield won't pay at least 80 percent of the purchase price of that truck?

22

"Did you check Cyclone's teeth, Doctor?"

OH, PLEASE don't hurt 'im!'' cried the lady. "Please don't hurt 'im!''

At least I thought that's what she was screaming.

I really couldn't hear her all that well because of the uproar being created by her horse and me.

It was one of those adopt-a-horse deals where some organization out west allows you to adopt a wild burro-like creature if you give it a good home, good feed and promise to supply it something to kick and bite every few days.

Another part of the deal is that the new owner must see to it that the good health of the animal is maintained, as much as possible. This is where the veterinarian frequently gets involved, and that is why I presently was involved in a major fracas with a fiesty burro by the name of Cyclone.

Because Cyclone's owner was terrified of him and getting close enough to halter the beast was out of the question, I was forced to bring out my lariat and rope him as if he were a rodeo steer. I knew it was going to be chaos.

Went beserk!

Sure enough, when the nylon cinched down on his neck, Cyclone went beserk. He absolutely exploded into a kicking, jumping, squealing and wheezing frenzy. Round and round the small corral we struggled while dust and debris were flying like confetti. With each lap around the pen, I took up slack in the line, and soon I was within striking distance of his flying hooves. Finally, I was dangerously close enough that I quickly injected a tranquilizer into his sweaty neck.

The prick of the needle was met with additional jumps, squeals and attempts to rearrange the mud, trash and sod of the corral. I was reeling backwards, trying to avoid the pawing hooves. That's when I heard the plea of the lady.

"Don't worry, ma'am," I replied, just two seconds after scrambling to safety, "he's not gonna get me!"

"Oh, I wasn't worried about you, Doctor," she allowed. "It's poor Cyclone. He's so precious and innocent."

Precious and innocent? Perhaps so, but I don't see how anything precious could be so intent on sending someone to intensive care or the mortuary.

Some minutes later, I completed the vaccinations and the deworming with minimal effort. Cyclone wasn't sedated sufficiently by any means, but he was a step slower which enabled me to ease up and get the injections done, then slip away before he could react. The deworming was a bigger problem, but with perseverance it finally was accomplished.

I quickly removed the rope and escaped over the plank fence onto the safety of the bermuda-grassed backyard. As I breathed a sigh of relief, I looked back into the corral to see ol' Cyclone lie down for a snooze. His eyes closed, and his tongue lolled out. He looked totally harmless.

"Did his teeth have any cavities, Doctor?" queried the lady.

I knew that I had very clearly heard what she had said, but I couldn't believe it!

"Ma'am? Did you say teeth? Cavities?"

"Yes, of course! Does he have good teeth? Any malocclusion?"

I was stunned! Never before had I heard such a question! I often had floated and filed off sharp equine teeth and had extracted a few diseased molars, but horse owners just aren't in the habit of inquiring about cavities, correct bites, or coffee stains.

"Well, uh, I really didn't look very closely at his teeth," I stammered. "But what I did see sure looked great!" I grinned, but she did not.

With teeth gritted and nostrils flared, I climbed back over into the pen and tiptoed up to the snoozing equine. I carefully examined his molars by palpating them through the skin on both sides of his face. They felt fine. Now, if I could just take a quick peek at his incisors and open up his mouth.

But, when I reached into the side of his oral cavity and grabbed his slimy tongue, he came unglued — again. This time I was holding onto his neck with my right arm while he went into his vet-shedding dance. After a few seconds of this routine, he suddenly stopped dead still, with his head up against a chinaberry tree. I quickly glanced at his incisors, released him and again jumped over the fence.

"Perfect teeth!" I announced to the lady. "If folks had teeth that good, all these dentists around here would go broke!" I laughed, but she did not. "How about his feet?" she asked.

I couldn't believe this! I just stood motionless for a few seconds while my temper index rose several notches.

"Where is this all going to end?" I thought to myself. "Next it'll be tonsils, then she'll want his eyes ophthalmoscoped, then we'll have to psychoanalyze him."

"Lady, let me make a suggestion," I said very slowly and calmly. "I am very busy today and I have several other calls to make, hopefully before dark. Also, I think I have risked my life enough today. So, if you don't mind, I will come again another day after you have fed Cyclone some tranquilizer powders, and I'll do a complete physical exam on him. Is that satisfactory?"

"Oh, I don't know," she said. "I just don't want anything to happen to him."

Call McDaniel . . .

"Tell you what let's do. I'll come back next week, but, in the meantime, if you want to call Dr. McDaniel in from over at Red Hill, that will be quite all right with me. He's a real horse expert, and I recommend him to you very highly!"

"Oh no!" she exclaimed, "We want you to be Cyclone's doctor. Our dairymen neighbors all say you're such a good vet, and you are a lot cheaper than Dr. McDaniel."

Since that day, my professional fees for doing horse work have increased substantially. I don't know of a single veterinarian who wants to be called "cheap," especially when vetting a wild horse.

The lady talked with Dr. McDaniel on the phone, but he was way too busy to help with her companion animal. He very graciously referred her back to me.

Therefore, I had a return engagement with Cyclone. The second time he reacted nicely to the tranquilizer that we put into his grain some hours before. I examined him from head to tip of his tail. When I finished I asked for advice.

"I've checked everything I can think of Ma'am," I announced, "Is there anything else you can think of?"

"Is he old enough to get married?" she asked. "If so, I am thinking of adopting him a wife."

"No, Ma'am, he's way too young for anything like that!" I lied seriously.

One Cyclone is enough!

23

There are several kinds of wavers

Do you know **everybody?**" asked the young veterinary student as we drove down the country road.

"I don't think so. Why?"

"Well, you wave at everybody you meet, and they all wave back."

"I suppose that's just another nice thing about being a country veterinarian," I replied.

"A lot of them are farmers and clients, so I either make calls to their place, know them from agricultural associations or just recognize their pickup trucks 'cause I've seen 'em parked at their houses."

It is true that waving to oncoming drivers is normal operating procedure for me. Perhaps this habit can be traced back to my boyhood days, when I observed my father and uncles doing the same thing.

"You ought to always speak," Dad always said. "It might be the banker!"

"Always wave at the police," Sam Pete Smith always said.

Sam Pete believed strongly that smiling broadly and waving with enthusiasm at "the law" would return dividends somewhere along the line.

From a business standpoint, Dad and Sam Pete were both correct. However, I believe that waving at oncoming vehicles tends to make both wavers feel a little better and the day a little more pleasant. It's kind of like when a friend unexpectedly treats you to a moon pie and pint of cold milk at a country store. It is a small gesture, but the small kindnesses often mean as much as the large ones.

In studying the waving phenomenon, I have concluded that there are four main types of waving techniques. Often you can accurately predict the personality of a waver, just by carefully noting his or her mannerisms.

Finger wave . . .

The finger wave is performed by holding one or both hands on top of the steering wheel, then raising one index finger as the wavee approaches. The finger can be raised and held in the upward position when the oncoming truck is a quarter of a mile away or it can be raised at the last moment, almost too late to be seen.

Finger wavers usually are grim-faced, no-nonsense type fellows who often drive Dodges or Internationals. Some can't see very well, so they hesitate because they don't want to be seen speaking to a bushy tree or to the lead hippie in a motorcycle gang. They eat vanilla ice cream.

I know a veterinarian or two who wave with fingers. They always are deep in thought, probably about how they're going to treat the next sick cow or how best to get a check out of a nonpaying client.

As a rule, finger wavers are hard to deal with. They don't tell jokes or like to listen to them, they smile at very little, and most of the ones I work with think I charge too much for my services. However, they always have their cows penned up and will pay their vet bill — even though they think it's too high!

Hand and arm waving is the most common kind of greeting I engage. A single throw up of the right hand and arm, accompanied by a moderate smile, is standard. These are the everyday kind of people who have the same problems that most folks have. They look forward to Monday night football on the TV, are pretty steady types and become properly enraged when "the gov'mint" is mentioned. They sometimes forget to do things like having the cows ready for the vet or paying the bill on time. They eat chocolate ice cream and are only occasionally adventurous enough to order strawberry.

Total body wave . . .

Total body wavers are a sight to behold. A few of my friends fit into this category. Usually, when the oncoming vehicles are as much as a half mile away, the total body waver goes into action. He blinks his lights on and off, veers his truck in and out of both lanes, honks his horn and takes both hands off the steering wheel. One hand is thrown outside the window, and the other is working rapidly back and forth on the inside of the windshield.

Sometimes a foot and leg can be observed jumping back and forth on the dash board. His mouth is open in a wide, moving grin, obviously shouting not just words, but entire paragraphs. In short, the guy seems to be experiencing a conniption fit, but miraculously the pickup truck remains in the confines of the proper lane, give or take six feet or so.

These people are fun, but scatter-brained types, who never remember vet check day but are so full of devilment and good cheer that it's hard to get angry at them. They always have a new joke to tell, know all the latest football gossip and are liable to order tutti-frutti or rum ball ice cream at the store.

Head nodders never are first to wave at anybody. However, when waved at, they react with a quick throwback of the head. The reason for this is that they are slow mentally. When they see someone waving, it takes a period of time for that to register in the wave control area of the brain. If they wait long enough for the brain to tell the finger or hand to move, they will be waving at the next vehicle.

I'm a little suspicious of head nodders because I'm never sure of whether they're slow, just unfriendly or the cow died. They don't eat ice cream unless force fed and only then if it's some off flavor type, such as peach.

In addition to the four main groups, there are several minor groups. There are the saluters, mostly older men who were sergeants in World War II or the Korean Conflict. When saluted, I find myself going rigid and saluting back. I dislike meeting these guys because it brings back unfond memories of paratrooper school at Fort Campbell.

The right hand over the left ear wave rarely is seen anymore. This wave, perfected by Mr. Frank Harlow, a Tennessee school bus driver, apparently is a lost art. I use it occasionally just to observe the puzzled looks I get.

The type waver you are really makes no difference, just as long as you wave. It will make you feel better, and it will help to build a better relationship between you and your neighbors. Besides, it might be the banker or the law.

24

Don't be so busy that you forget to look

IT WAS Saturday morning and the clinic was a madhouse. The waiting room was crammed full of people with dogs, cats and a gerbil, while the parking lot contained two or three pickup trucks and trailers containing an assortment of livestock. The phone was ringing constantly, and the two-way radio was picking up interesting skips of messages from far off places.

Each spring, staticky conversations bounced over our radio from veterinarians in places like Black River Falls, Wis.; Princeton, Ill.; Athens, Ohio; Bedford, Pa.; and Texas A&M Veterinary School.

That morning, Dr. Hart in Wisconsin sounded busy, too, since his wife already had radioed two milk fevers, a prolapsed uterus and a calf delivery to him in the last hour.

While Jan was writing up a ticket, I grabbed the ringing phone. It was a hog farmer with a request for service.

"Doc, I'm gonna send one of my boys down there with an old Duroc boar that I want you to cut," he said.

"Fine, send him on down in about an hour," I suggested.

When I hung up, Jan told me about another hog that was coming in.

"Tobe Landrum is sending one of his boys up here with a purebred Duroc boar to be tested for Bang's and pseudorabies," she stated, as we passed in the waiting room.

I immediately thought of a near tragic boar hog mixup that had befallen Dr. Robinson, one of my colleagues in a nearby town. He and his receptionist both had received the exact type calls that Jan and I had received that morning. He, too, was busy, running from case to case, trying to finish up at the clinic in order to get going on his farm calls.

When a pickup truck pulled into the driveway, Dr.

Robinson had grabbed his instrument tray, hog snare, anesthetic agent, other hog castrating paraphernalia and quickly jogged out to the patient. He jumped over into the truck, snared the boar's nose and handed it to the young lad to hold. He quickly injected the drug into the ear vein and presently the patient was sleeping soundly.

The young lad apparently didn't understand what was happening until the surgical site had been scrubbed and the Doctor had pulled on surgical gloves. Just as the scalpel made a four-inch incision, however, the young man suddenly came alive.

"No, No!" he screamed. Then, just as quickly, he fainted, collapsing head first into the tray of instruments and onto a stainless steel bucket.

Naturally, human injuries take priority over veterinary matters in such situations. Removing his gloves and calling for help from bystanders, Dr. Robinson and the others soon had the bleeding, moaning and wall-eyed youngster moved into the waiting room and onto the sofa. Cold towels applied to his face quickly brought him back to consciousness.

"What happened, Son?" asked the Doctor.

"Uh, Daddy just wanted that boar blood-tested," he stammered slowly.

"He just paid $1,000 for him up in Illinois. When you started to cut on 'im, I reckon I just fainted. Daddy would've skint me an' you both if you'd have cut that high-price boar!"

"Why didn't you speak up before I cut?"

"Well, I figured you knowed what you was doin' till you picked up that knife."

It was said that Dr. Robinson had to lay down with the boy and put cold towels on his face to keep from fainting.

After a short rest, the young boy was taken to the hospital for head stitches while Dr. Robinson went back out to the truck and put stitches in the other end of the boar. While suturing the prize boar, a truck drove up carrying the hog for which the surgery was intended.

I giggled to myself, thinking of how we all make such dumb mistakes, in spite of trying to keep things going on an even keel. As I ran outside, Willie Franklin caught me.

"Doc, how 'bout vaccinatin' those two Holsteins over

there for Bang's or whatever they need," he exclaimed.

"Sure, Willie," I said, "why don't you halter 'em while I get my tagging pliers."

Steers vaccinated . . .

In minutes I had given both the Bang's vaccine, as well as blackleg, IBR and BVD — the usual shots. Then I put the orange tag in their right ears and applied the proper tattoo. As I was writing up the calfhood vaccination record, Willie asked another question.

"Doc, would you check and be sure they're both steers?"

I was writing furiously, but when I hear the word "steers," I stopped recording ear tag numbers in midscribble.

"Steers? Did you say steers?" I said softly, "I thought you said they were heifers!"

"I never said they wuz heifers!" he yelled. "I thought every vet knew the difference 'twixt a steer and a heifer, but apparently I was mistaken!"

Sure enough, when I looked they were both steers. I just shook my head at my stupidity and tore the vaccination record in half.

Although it may not be common knowledge among the noncattle, owning public, Bang's vaccine is to be given only to calves of the female variety. It is a definite "no-no" to vaccinate a bull or steer against this disease. The "feds" won't allow male cattle to receive the vaccine; nor will they accept a certificate of vaccination indicating such. As a matter of fact, they probably would become somewhat riled if someone did such a thing and then made the mistake of reporting it.

Over the years, I have come in contact with hundreds of veterinarians from all over the world. None of them have owned up to ever vaccinating a bull or steer against Bang's disease. Something tells me that some of them are lying through their teeth!

This mistake brings to mind a truism frequently uttered by my professor colleague, Dr. Dilmus Blackmon.

"You miss a lot more by not looking than by not knowing."

This is good advice for everybody but especially for veterinarians!

25

Domineckers and the silver cow

LIKE most large animal practitioners, I don't really mind working on Christmas Day, if it's necessary. I do mind leaving my family to carry out routine procedures that should have been done earlier or could be put off until the first week of January. Things such as boar hog castrations, umbilical hernia repairs or mange treatments easily can be scheduled another time.

Its the borderline stuff that causes me problems. Metritis cases, foot abscesses, displaced abomasums and semen tests all seem like things that could wait at least until Santa Claus has exited the county.

So when the lady called Christmas Eve wanting information about retained placentas in cows, I was less than enthusiastic.

"We usually don't treat them until 72 hours after calving unless the cow appears sick," I told her. "When did she calve?"

"Oh, about ten days ago," she replied.

"Ten days ago! Is she sick?"

"Oh yes, she won't eat, droops around real bad, and spends most of her time lying down," she replied.

"Yeah, I'll bet she does," I sighed.

Now the question. "Should I go on out tonight or should I wait and go in the morning?" I asked myself.

"Do you have her penned up?" was the obvious next question.

"No, she's out in the pasture." That's what I figured.

"If you'll get her into a pen or the barn, I'll come on out right now and take care of her before dark," I replied. I scribbled down directions to the farm and was soon on my way.

Some 20 miles, a double handful of Jan's Christmas candy and a pint of milk later, I wheeled in between the two broiler houses at the end of the gravel road, crossed the gap and stopped in front of an old barn. Just like the directions read.

Mrs. Puckett, the calling lady, was off to the right side of the house washing a brand new pickup truck with an old rag, a stew pot of water and what appeared to be a bar of motel soap. She was wearing a bonnet, an old timey housewife smock, and sturdy oxford shoes, substantial enough for steel mill work. The truck was long as a school bus, with every gadget and option available. I'm sure it must have cost $20,000.

I was struck by the contrasts of the modern truck being motel soap-hand washed by a lady in such old-fashioned garb.

"Cow's over yonder," she yelled, pointing to the other side of an old log barn.

Now I have seen bovines penned in corrals, barns, smokehouses, back porches and bread trucks up on blocks, but I had never before seen a cow penned up with hens in a glorified chicken coop.

But there she was, standing underneath a row of six hen nests, two of which contained hens. The other nests contained "nest eggs," which actually were old white door knobs. I reckon these door knobs fool the hens into getting up in the nest and laying an egg while trying to incubate and meditate over the door knob.

The dozen or so nervous fowl were of the "Dominecker" variety. Carney Sam Jenkins, homemade veterinarian and gifted seer, always called them "Barred Rock Beauties." They are kind of guinea colored, gray with large white specks. They are known to be good layers, good setters, and they'll eat you alive when they have biddies under their wings.

I also found out that evening that those Domineckers don't care much for the presence of a bovine in their nesting area. They were clucking around, jerking their heads about in crazy chicken fashion, seemingly quizzing each other about the large silvery beast slowly moving around in their midst.

The cow was the color of a schnauzer, and she had the odor of rotten kraut. I insisted, with kind words, that she move out of the coop into the triangular corner of the wire "patio," but she refused. I needed to push on her rear parts, but due to her present state of personal hygiene, I was unenthusiastic about such an assist.

By that time Mr. Puckett, a wimpy looking fellow, had shuffled over, grabbed the top strand of the chicken wire fence and was sort of hanging there, observing the carryings on. I popped the stinking beast on the behind with my rope and she jumped out of the hen house door, with several Domineckers running, flying and squawking immediately preceding her.

"Don't hurt my hens!" the man pleaded. "You're scaring my hens, feller!"

The cow had her head lowered and eyes closed as she charged into the narrow corner. The dozen or so hens also were charging into the same corner, and they were getting stomped and thrashed about as they chaotically flew and flopped into the fence, their eyes the size of dimes. Dust, debris and feathers were flying like confetti, the fence squawked each time a panicking hen flew into it and two recently arrived mangy dogs began barking and biting into the battered fence, trying to secure a Christmas meal of very rare poultry fricassee.

I was yelling at the dogs and Mr. Puckett was yelling at me, while I was trying to keep the cow shoved into the corner, all the time waving the rope in the general direction of her head. Out of nowhere Mrs. Puckett appeared, and with one swift kick of her right brogan oxford, she dispatched the dogs toward the house, slinking and whining through the pines.

Mr. Puckett also slinked quietly toward the house, the look on his face indicating he was sure he was the next victim. Then she glared at me, but I was involved getting the loop tight around the cow's neck and the other end tied to a nearby post.

I learned many years ago that when things in the corral get turbulent, it is time to send someone to the house for warm water. Now was the time for such a request.

"Mrs. Puckett, would you please run to the house and get me a bucket of water?" I requested, out-voicing both poultry and cow.

"Gladly," she allowed, with hand over her face, "anything to get away from this stinking cow!''

Once the cow was secured, I commenced catching the hens that had become trapped in the corner. I was grabbing wings, legs, necks, or any other feathery handle available and tossing them back toward the henhouse. Some were hung in the fence, and extracting them took two hands.

Unfortunately, the 1,000-pound bovine patient was terrified of all the noise and rushing wind created by the flopping, seven-pound birds. She exhibited her anxiety by pulling back on the rope almost to the point of choking, all the while peering at the poultry.

Suddenly, rasping and wheezing, the cow collapsed with a thud, narrowly missing a chunky Dominecker. I quickly gave the rope around her neck a foot of slack and continued removing the poultry remaining from in the area.

While the patient was regaining her wits and her breath, I noticed that the decaying afterbirth was now hanging out much further than before all the chaos began. When she started to sit up, I stomped my boot on the thing and as she rose, all ten pounds of it slid right out, as slick as a whistle.

A quick glance toward the house revealed there was no one in sight, not even the disgruntled dogs, so I drew some antibiotic and hormone into a couple of syringes, and had the patient injected and released by the time the lady arrived fenceside with a five-gallon grease bucket full of boiling water.

''You finished already?'' she puffed, obviously semi-exhausted from lugging the vat of water. Now she had her smock up over her nose in mask-like fashion.

''Yes Ma'am, getting that nasty thing out nearly whipped us both!'' I exclaimed, kicking the recently removed specimen closer to the fence for her inspection. The lady jumped back as if she had just seen a copperhead.

Meanwhile, the cow had re-entered the narrow egg laying area and was again terrorizing the Domineckers. Mrs. Puckett produced a claw hammer from somewhere under her clothes and with a few pulls and jerks soon had the fence half down. The cow was soon in the pasture and was vigorously grabbing mouthfuls of fescue.

''Why just look at her!'' she exclaimed. ''She feels better already.''

"Yes, Ma'am. Isn't science wonderful," I replied, tongue in cheek and fingers crossed. I commenced washing my hands and arms vigorously in the scalding water. "Never ask a farmer for *hot* water!" I reminded myself.

"If you'll drive back up to the house, I'll write you a check," she allowed.

Once at the house, I noticed the DVM sticker on the rear bumper of the spotless new truck.

"Sure is a nice truck, you got here," I said.

"Oh yes, that belongs to my son. He's a vet, too, from Atlanta."

"Why didn't he doctor on the cow for you?" I asked.

"Oh no, he's a small animal practitioner. They told him in school there was no challenge or future in large animals. He makes good money working nights in an emergency clinic," she declared as she signed the check and handed it over. "Besides, it's Christmas, and I couldn't ask him to do something like that when he's off."

"Yes, Ma'am."

"Well, that sure is a lot to pay to get a cow cleaned off," she sighed, handing over the check. "Maybe I should have awakened my son and got him to do it."

"No, Ma'am, I wouldn't do that, there's no future in it. Besides, it takes a special skill to do what I did," I declared, again with fingers crossed and tongue in cheek.

I'm sure that young vet enjoys working nights in a big city emergency animal clinic as much as I enjoy working with cows and their owners. Isn't it great that every veterinarian doesn't like the same thing?

26

I remember hoecakes and a six teated cow

ONE of childhood's great privileges is being routinely exposed to one's aunts and uncles. I firmly believe that their influence on a youngster frequently rivals that of the natural parents. I was very fortunate to have been issued a fine set of relatives, all of whom have exerted positive impressions upon my life.

The majority of my ancestors have been farmers. Since they milked cows, raised sheep and swine, grew tobacco, corn, wheat and hay, they were classified as "general farmers." It was a good way to farm, and sometimes I wonder if farmers and society in general wouldn't be better off if things still were done that way.

One good thing about having relatives nearby was that I had the opportunity to visit, sometimes spending entire weeks with them during haying season when I could be spared from home.

During these visits, I was just like a regular family member or hired man when it came to doing routine chores. If we were baling hay, for instance, I still was expected to help feed the hens, slop the hogs, pick string beans and milk the cows. I might even wheelbarrow the full milk cans out to the road where the Bordens, Kraft or Ardmore Creamery milk truck would pick them up.

Aunt Nannie and Uncle Robert had no children of their own, but to them all the flock of nieces and nephews were like their own. And, we especially enjoyed being there since we were allowed to do things for which we probably would have been thrashed had we been at home. There always was a cookie jar full of tea cakes as big as strainer pads, to which we had free and easy access. We smugly drank coffee, heavily diluted with milk retrieved not from a refrigerator but from a cool spring behind the barn.

As special as "white coffee" was, it was not nearly as special as those hot water hoecakes that Aunt Nannie cooked in her special black skillet. I doubt that the cuisine at a fancy restaurant in Paris or Hong Kong could compare with that early morning hoecake, especially after it had been liberally smeared with butter; real butter, not that no-taste oleo that looks like jaundiced lard.

At milking time, we gathered Borden buckets and the strainer before heading for the barn. As we walked, we called the cows.

"Whew, suk, suk, suk, suk!" we yelled in the direction of the pasture, cupping our hands, megaphone-like around our mouths.

This "suk, suk!" jargon is cow talk for "come on down here to this barn! Right now!" It never dawned on me how to spell the work "suk" until one day when a young veterinary student from New York City asked me how to spell it. I was confused and still don't know the proper spelling.

If pasture was succulent and green, the cows dawdled until someone, usually a small boy or a clever dog, trudged up the path and retrieved them. If pasture was short, dried up, or dense with bitterweed, the bovines usually would be waiting at the gate.

It wasn't uncommon to do the milking outside the barn or wherever the cow stopped. A treat of cottonseed hulls, crushed corn and cottonseed meal was presented to the milkee, while the milker went to work. It was important to milk fast, with both hands, in order to finish before the feed bucket had been licked clean and the cow commenced sauntering around the lot. I have seen cows actually being milked in the middle of the public gravel road. Passersby, unless aggressive, would have to stop and wait.

Healthy head of foam . . .

People who are good hand milkers have a minor problem with foam. The turbulence created by two profuse and brisk streams of milk also produces lots of foam atop the rising level of milk. Therefore, there soon may be more inches of foam than inches of milk. I doubt if it would make much sense to youngsters today, but when I finally was able to milk a healthy head of foam onto a bucket of milk, I knew that I was on my way to becoming a grown-up.

The cows that were assigned to me were those easiest to milk. They had odd names, such as Newman, Model T, One Horn or Hedgeapple. But the one that I especially remember was called Six Teat. This half Shorthorn marvel possessed six teats, all of which produced milk. The rear two naturally were shorter, but still could be milked without great effort. She also was a slow eater which was handy, since it took longer to milk six teats that it did four.

Milking would not be done in silence. In between the sounds of sheep bleating, a donkey braying a mile away, and the buzzing of July flies in the maple trees, Aunt Nannie and Uncle Robert would be carrying on a conversation about the daily farming activities. Sometimes the private life of the nephew would be investigated.

"How many girl friends you have, John?" my uncle teased.

"None, I reckon," I replied.

"Aw come on! I heard there was a little girl in Elkton who helped you hoe corn last week!"

"No, Sir, she came over with her mother to buy some eggs and butter," I said. "I think she just came out in the field to see what I was doing."

After the girl friend dialogue had been exhausted, the talk would drift toward laying by the corn, what the news was from the monthly missionary society meeting and who had been seen driving up into the hollow that day.

"Saw cow! Saw now!" someone would occasionally bark.

For the uninformed, the word "saw" was directed to the cow. It means for the cow to cease her sashaying at once and be still! I am not at all sure of it's proper spelling either. How to spell "saw" never occurred to me until a student from Miami asked.

Every few minutes the sound of six streams of milk being squirted into the three buckets was reduced to four. Seconds later the familiar tinkle of metal indicated that the rich milk was being poured from bucket into strainer. As the milk drained into the dented can, the young lad would be wondering how heavy the wheelbarrow was going to roll that night when he pushed it the quarter mile to the public road.

Straining the milk was important, and my folks always used a Kendall six-and-a-half inch strainer pad, not a clean fertilizer sack like some people. Besides, a milk-soaked strainer pad was a greatly coveted postmilking snack for the family dog, who ingested it with gusto. It was odd, though, how that dog always exhibited a wheezing attack immediately after swallowing the pad. It was as if he had inhaled a large dip of smokeless tobacco.

Sometimes, when the days became short, the late barn chores were done by kerosene lantern light since there was no electricity. As we marched down the path to the house, the swinging lantern and human legs cast eerie shadows on the ground. A good imagination could conjure up all sorts of weird creatures that the shadows represented.

Back in the house, the kerosene lamp was lit, a cold supper of noontime leftovers was consumed and perhaps a carefully selected program was enjoyed on the battery radio. Just before bed time, a passage was read from the Bible, and prayers were said. Then it was off to bed so we could arise early and do it all over again.

Times were hard, and so was the work. But I keep wondering if we weren't just as well off then as we are today. It seems that there weren't nearly as many psycological or physical problems back then. Perhaps it was because of those good hoecakes and home-churned butter, along with plenty of outside exercise. However, in spite of all that, I don't want to go back to those days.

Just a few days ago, many of those nieces and nephews met at Uncle Robert and Aunt Nannie's farmhouse to celebrate her 79th birthday. As we stepped out of the pickup truck and started up the walkway, my keen sense of smell picked up a wonderful kitchen aroma I remembered from long ago. Suddenly I was a kid again.

"Got you a hoecake on the stove, Johnny Boy!" quipped a smiling Aunt Nannie as she gave me a big hug. It tasted as good as I recalled.

I should have gone out to the old barn, with buttered hoecake in hand, to see if the ghost of old Six Teat still roams the barn lot!

27

"You have razor bran for breakfast?"

Doc, this red bull of mine has a big knot on his side," the early-morning caller allowed.

Actually, it was real early. I was awake but had not yet crawled out of bed on that Monday morning. My mind was reviewing the schedule for the day and wondering how many additional calls would come in. I was hoping that I could make the cattlemen's meeting that night.

"Well, that's an oddball thing," I replied, sarcastically. "They always told me that knots were on trees but bulls had swellings or abscesses. Better call the newspaper!"

"Boy, you're sharp this morning, ain't you," he said. "You have razor bran for breakfast? Reckon you're sharp enough to cure this swelling, or have I got to find a veterinarian?"

The caller was Woodson Montgomery, one of my livestock-owning neighbors and one of the best farmers in the county. We have been good friends for many years, and I have been an invited guest in his corrals, pastures and barns on many occasions.

Regardless of whether it's a phone call or a trip to the farm, Woodson and his associates, Shelnutt and Choice, always are ready with good-natured kidding and are armed with a plethora of verbal barbs.

They have made jokes about my ineptness with a lariat, just because I had some difficulty one time when trying to rope a crippled calf. After about six throws, I finally caught the beast by the left foreleg. Since that time, no call that I make to the farm is complete without some sarcastic reference to the calf-roping episode.

Another item that seldom escapes being discussed is the encounter I had with a small calf several years ago. The 200-pound bull calf looked gentle and friendly, but, when I wrestled him down in order to examine his swollen navel, he exploded into a kicking frenzy. Of course, no one offered assistance because they were all too busy doubled up splitting their sides with laughter. Meanwhile, the bottom of the poor beast's little hooves were being tattooed repeatedly to my arms, shoulders and the side of my head.

"Here's one about your speed, Doc," Shelnutt had allowed one day, pointing to a 24-hour-old, 60-pound Angus. "Reckon you can git the best of him?"

All I could do was stare with contempt. If a look could have caused trauma, Shelnutt would have had to be transported to intensive care for at least a week.

I arrived at the barn right after lunch to see the bull with the knot on his side. No one was around, and all was quiet except for the sound of my patient's lips as he chewed his cud with enjoyment. He looked at me curiously but never missed a chew. Finally, he stopped, swallowed, then paused for a few seconds. Suddenly, I saw the outline of a new cud as it traveled in reverse back up his neck and into his big mouth. He commenced chewing immediately.

Sometimes when I have spare time I just sit or stand quietly and watch cows chew their cuds and marvel at these amazing creatures. Their ability to graze and grow on grasses, forages and other almost useless products from land unsuitable for anything else is a physiological miracle. The resulting milk and meat are without a doubt the two finest foods consumed by man.

"How many times does a cow chew her cud before she swallows it?" my dad asked me many years ago.

Chewed 52 times . . .

Since then I frequently have counted the chews. Woodson's red bull chewed one cud 52 times before he sent it back down his gullet.

Getting back to business, I saw the swelling on the left side of the bull. It was about at the level of his elbow, in the region of the ninth rib. Not a rare place for an abscess, but a little unusual.

He went into the chute real nice, and I put a locust post behind him before catching his head. As I was palpating the soft mass, Woodson came walking slowly from the house. From the look of his eyes, it was obvious he had been taking an after-dinner nap.

"Oh, did I disturb your beauty nap?" I said softly. "Next time I'll try to make less racket. After all, I wouldn't want you to have to wake up just to help me!"

He sneered, yawned and sat down on an upside-down bucket.

"What is it?" he said.

"An abscess," I replied.

"How come?"

"Don't know."

"Whatcha gon' do?"

"Lance it."

"Will it heal up?"

"Yep."

With the conversation out of the way, I scrubbed and shaved a small area where the swelling was softest, then quickly stuck it with a needle to be sure it was what I thought it was. Sure enough, dirty yellow pus dripped out the needle.

Next, I quickly made a stab incision with a scalpel and just as quickly enlarged the incision. About a gallon of pus, blood and gunk flowed out.

"Man, that's nasty," said Choice, who had just sauntered up. He'd been napping, too.

"I coulda done that," allowed Woodson, "and saved this call."

"Well, why didn't you?" I replied, while packing the abscess cavity with a roll of iodined gauze. "I sure got plenty else to do."

"I figured you needed the practice," he said.

"Naw, I just need the money. And I like coming to these rich turkey and cow farmers 'cause I know they got plenty of it."

"Shoot!" he exclaimed. "I'm so broke I can't even pay attention!"

A few weeks later I stopped by Woodson's sweet corn field to get a sack full of roasting ears. While there, I heard Woodson's truck pull up behind mine. Presently, we met in between the corn rows.

"What you doin' in my corn patch, Boy?" he yelled.

"Just checking for disease in these nubbins," I allowed. "Got to confiscate a few dozen ears, take 'em to the lab and get 'em checked. Looks like worms!"

"Bout that bull, Doc. His side is swollen back up worse than ever!"

"Uh oh!" I said. "Let's go see about it right now."

Recurring abscesses frequently mean that a foreign body is present somewhere in the mass. That's what I told Woodson after checking it the second time.

"When I lance this thing, I'm gonna find a piece of baling wire down in there, about four or five inches long with a crook on the other end."

Sure enough, after I had drained the pus and flushed the cavity, my gloved finger felt the tip of something sharp. Exploring with a pair of long-handled forceps, I finally extracted a four-inch piece of wire with the crook on one end.

As I held it high for viewing, Woodson, Choice and Shelnutt all came up close for inspection of the foreign body. foreign body.

"What do you think of that?" I questioned proudly. I thought they would be impressed with my great predicting ability and my skill as a bull surgeon.

"It took two expensive trips to find a piece of baling wire?" one asked.

"You're not so smart, Doc," allowed Shelnutt. "You said the crook was gonna be on the other end of that wire!"

Now that crowd has something else to pick on me about. How could I have known that the crook would be on the other end of that wire?

Sometimes good friends have odd ways of cultivating and maintaining their friendships. However, those often are the first ones to help you out when your ox gets in a ditch or the creek gets out of banks.

28

Brain overload causes loss of memory

IT'S getting worse. I've always had a problem losing things, but I didn't realize how serious the problem was until last week. Somehow I lost a large check from one of my clients, and it caused me to reflect on all the other things I've lost over the years.

Some say misplacing stuff is just carelessness; others say it is a sign of feeblemindedness, and still others declare that it's a sign of brain overload. That is to say that there are just too many things to think about and do which cause the brain waves to get short circuited or crossed up. The end result, simply, is a brain blackout concerning where he or she dropped the hoof knife, mislaid the dehorners or loaned out the jumper cables.

Times have changed so much and life has become so complex, it's no wonder that forgetfulness is plaguing so many individuals. In simpler times, the main things folks had to worry about were their next meal and watching out for a monster on the horizon. There were no truck payments, outrageous tax bills, television sets to buy or fishing trips to Canada just begging to be taken.

In addition, there weren't all these people around whose names and statistics had to be remembered. Zip codes, phone numbers, charge card code numbers and license tag figures are just a few of the likewise unheard of nuisances.

Want 'em back . . .

The following is a partial summary of items I have misplaced, lost or, in many instances, have been inadvertently left at farms. I would like to have them back.

Pocket knives of all descriptions are out there somewhere! There is a two-bladed, bone-handled Case somewhere near the Mississippi River levee down in Louisiana.

There's a three-bladed Buck somewhere in Georgia, a Boker Tree Brand in Choctaw County, Alabama, and a yellow-handled Schrade in Reno. The Schrade probably is in a pawn shop, along with some unlucky gambler's shirt, shoes and his poor wife's wedding ring.

"Honey, if all the knives you've lost were laid end to end, they'd reach from here to Michigan," Jan once said.

"Well, do you think I lose 'em on purpose?" I replied. "I do work with them, you know. I don't tote 'em around just to be socially acceptable." Well, maybe I do just a little. After all, what kind of person doesn't have a pocket knife?

I lost a real nice Case XX hunting knife and its sheath several years ago. This knife was one of my most prized possessions. Ten years later, one of my hunting buddies found it stuck up on a ceiling joist at Rudder Hill Hunting Club. He immediately recognized my mark on the scabbard and, being the honest, upright citizen that he is, obtained my address and sent it to me. I was overjoyed but within two weeks had lost it again, probably somewhere in my closet or perhaps in the woods behind the house.

Hoof knives and other devices used for cutting on cow feet are other items that I lose frequently. It's easy to drop these things in muck and straw when attempting to hold up a 1,500-pound cow's foot and pare out an abscess while trying to explain it to a bored dairyman sitting comfortably with his legs crossed, at a safe, no-work distance.

I think I missed that day at school, or wasn't paying close enough attention, when some clean, white-smocked professor must have explained how to do all this without dropping your knife. Of course, if we lived in more sensible times, there wouldn't be so many lame and sore-footed cows.

If consumers didn't demand such inexpensive food, then dairy farmers wouldn't be forced to put their cows on concrete and stuff 'em with so much grain and highly acid feeds. The end result would be cows with healthier hooves, thus less sole abscesses, ulcers and bruises. Then I'd need fewer aspirin tablets and extra strength BC powders, as well as knives.

Rope halters and nose tongs are the worst! I figure that I lose three halters a year, so in 30 years I have lost at least 90 of the things. Actually, I didn't lose all of them, I just left them at farms. What happens to them after that, I don't know, except that those farmers think the halters become the property of that farm. Sort of a "finders keepers, losers weepers" kind of thing.

Dyed my halter . . .

I know of one tricky cattleman who took one of my green-colored rope halters to the house and got his wife to dye it black. He bragged about it one night when he had a few too many helpings of white lightnin' after a cattlemen's meeting. I'll bet that happens more than I have realized. I've switched to a yellow color now, and I believe that this bright color is helpful when gathering up veterinary paraphernalia; makes it harder to miss when it's lying there in front of the chute or in the manger.

Dehorners, calf jacks, various surgical instruments and rubber boots are easily losable items. One veterinarian I know forgot where he left his portable squeeze chute and an absent-minded veterinary school Ph.D. professor once couldn't remember for a week where he had parked his old jalopy. The first day he couldn't recall whether or not he had driven it to work that morning. Some people are just educated beyond practical intelligence.

Today, I lost the keys to my pickup truck and had to crawl up under the thing to retrieve the spare set I wired to the frame for just such an emergency. For a moment I couldn't remember where I had hidden them.

The next problem I have is getting into my office in the morning, since that key also is lost. My house key and several other important keys also are on the ring. If and when I find them, I'm going to chain them to my belt loop.

To help prevent my losing so many things, I started taking a technician with me on calls. Her primary duty was to gather up all the equipment when we finished with the herd work. All went well until I forgot and left her at a dairy farm one day. After that episode, she quit.

I have come upon a possible solution to this loss of memory problem. I have decided to take a short course on improving things like name retention, prevention of personal item loss and stimulation of memory centers. As soon as I remember where I put the forms and questionnaire, I'll get right on it.

29

"I'm glad I'm not a chicken catcher"

OCCASIONALLY, the newspapers print some thought provoking and at least partially true articles. Just this past week, for instance, there was a story about the best and worst jobs in the U.S. These jobs were determined by evaluating them on the basis of salary, stress, work environment, outlook, severity and physical demands.

The good ones were all sit down kind of vocations like computer programmers, mathematicians, statisticians and actuaries. Actually, I didn't even know what an actuary was until I looked it up and found that it has to do with figuring how much to raise insurance premiums every few months. How hard can that be? All you have to do is get a cheap calculator and add 10 percent to all insurance premiums every six months. I reckon it is an easy job, unless there has been a claim. In that case, he or she adds on 20 percent or more, depending on how stressful the ride in had been that morning.

If his favorite country music station played only old Elvis tunes instead of the latest Don Williams or Randy Travis songs, that stressful situation could lead to increased insurance costs for the innocent consumer victims. All this is just dirt road theory, of course, but I think my suppositions are fairly close on target.

Is mathematics actually fun? Somehow I wonder whether a guy sitting at his desk ciphering and figuring all day, every day, for 20 to 30 years would be completely right. I know that after balancing the checkbook or doing the taxes, I sometimes just gallop out into the woods and bite tree bark in between yells.

I will agree that those jobs identified as "good jobs" don't require heavy lifting and working in the hot sun, so perhaps that is another reason they were chosen. Nor do they require much decision making or meeting of regular people.

The "worst job" list was equally interesting, but not totally surprising. The worst job of all, according to the authors, was that of migrant farmworker, preceded by fisherman and construction worker. I can understand the migrant worker selection, but fisherman puzzles me. I know at least one mathematician who retired at age 60 and now tries to catch fish every day. Whenever he catches a nice fish, he talks to it in an unknown tongue and giggles in an incoherent fashion. Then he turns the thing loose and tries to catch it or an identical one again.

Dairy farmer was sixth from the bottom and the profession of cowboying was only three steps above dairying in desirability. I think it is remarkable that the producers of the two finest foods known, milk and beef, were banished to the bottom of the list.

I have thought about this list a lot the last few days and I want to create my own good and bad list. I am just as qualified to do this as any other living person and my list is just as publishable as the next person's. Consider the following as my candidates for the five "least desirable" jobs.

1. **Chicken catcher:** Have you ever wondered about this job and what the average working life span of a chicken catcher is? It is measured in hours, not days or years.

Can you imagine pulling up to a dark chicken house about 9 p.m., putting on a mask and then wading in amongst 20,000 broilers, knowing that way before daylight they all will have to be leg grabbed and stuffed in crates? Just thinking about it makes me want to bite bark!

The dust, the flopping wings, the boredom and never being able to really enjoy the sight of a nice flock of chickens are additional disadvantages of this job.

2. **Barber:** How would you like to stand on your feet all day long, six days a week and entertain your customer, as well as all those waiting to be clipped. A good barber must know everything about everybody, plus must be an accomplished liar, political analyst, psychologist, medical consultant, historian and weather forecaster. Ask him any question about any subject and he will give you an answer.

"How much is Class I milk bringing in Marlette,

Michigan?" someone might ask, for example.

"Twenty dollars," he might answer. Never mind that he's wrong, since nobody in the shop has the foggiest notion anyway.

A barber must have a lot of gall and excellent hand-mouth coordination. It takes steady fingers and good nerves to trim close around a feller's ear without amputating it, while explaining the Middle East crisis to a group of people who think Iraq is an insurance company up north. That's why I think barbers are born, not made.

3. **Miner:** What can I say. I once went down into a coal mine and I haven't been right since. Even so, every person alive should be forced, sometime in their life, to participate in a dozen or so real tough activities. Such things as cleaning out hen houses, cutting off thorny fencerows and going down into a coal mine.

It's close down in there, also eerie and cold. Water is dripping and you can hear weird sounds coming from strange places. The seam of coal may be only 18 inches high which means that all work has to be done lying down. This kind of environment is right stressful, as well as potentially dangerous.

I suppose the reason I'm so afraid of close places is because of the time I crawled under a corn crib to investigate an old setting hen and proceeded to get hung between the floor joists and the ground. I don't remember how I got out of there, but ever since, I have been uncomfortable when boarding an elevator, changing oil in the truck or walking around the base of a freshly filled silo. There are a lot of other people who feel the same way.

4. **Pickup truck repossessor:** Can you imagine going back up in the hollow to a typical redneck or roughneck and telling him that you have come to take his beloved four-wheel drive back to the bank because he is way behind with his payments? Items inside the cab include his favorite deer rifle, all his Hank Williams, Jr., cassette tapes and his favorite mini spittoon. Do you think this is going to be pleasant? Multiply this a couple of hundred times and you get an idea of what this job is like. I suspect the average lifespan of a truck repossessor is about the equivalent of a machine gunner on Iwo Jima.

5. **Spouse of a large animal veterinarian:** This is a life of

filthy coveralls, green-stained tee shirts, tracked up carpets and vehicles that smell strange.

"What's that peculiar odor in your station wagon?" a guest rider might inquire.

"Uh, what odor?" the spouse is sure to reply.

"Don't you smell that pungent . . ."

"Oh, that must be Bag Balm and B vitamins. Plus I've got two OB sleeves full of necropsy samples in the trunk that we've got to drop off at the diagnostic lab." A feeling of nausea may suddenly wave over the stomach of the guest rider at this point. Therefore, it is prudent to have anticipated this and have an emergency stopping place in mind.

Sometimes the kids and their playmates find odd things in cracks and crevices of the car.

"What's this, mister?" a neighborhood child might ask while holding up a device.

"Uh, it's just a speculum," the spouse might say.

"What's it for?"

"To use on cows."

"Take that nasty thing out of your mouth this instant, Junior!" is the quick response from the parent in the front seat. "There's no telling where it's been!"

Some spouses seem to be embarrassed by this kind of scene. I don't understand why!

It is obvious that everyone may not share my opinions about these so-called "undesirable" jobs. Some people seem to enjoy some of them.

I remember a guy back home who claimed he loved to clean out the hen house. Once a week, he'd get his hoe, shovel and wheel barrow together and head for that henhouse. On the way by the tractor shed, he'd get some used crankcase oil to pour over the mite-infested roosts.

We could hear him whistling and singing hymns while he scraped and shoveled. All went well until the day he finally snapped and started catching all the hens and stuffing them into crates. He confessed that he'd always had a secret hankering to be a professional chicken catcher. His poor family eventually sent him to the asylum where he studied barbering. Unfortunately, he didn't get much in-mate business because they figured anybody who enjoyed cleaning out hen houses and catching chickens was insane.

30

Good jobs are hard to come by

IT IS risky business to make lists and descriptions of the worst and best jobs in the world. After all, who is truly qualified to make such a determination? What it comes down to is that a listing can be made by just about anybody, such as a social worker, a journalist, a milk truck driver, an unemployed welder or, in this case, a veterinarian.

A good job, in my opinion, must have several positive features and a minimum of negative ones. It should be challenging to the mind and body, rewarding both financially and spiritually, and there should be a good reason for it to exist in the first place. Also, the best jobs produce a product or deliver a service that everybody wants or desperately needs.

The people or other creatures to be worked with also should be productive types, possess a sense of humor and be pleasant to be around. Some physical and mental stress is inevitable in every job, but there shouldn't be some arrogant supervisor sitting behind a clean desk thinking up ways to harrass and stress the people who do all the work. With these thoughts in mind, I have selected the five jobs that I think are the best.

1. **Pickup truck salesman:** I have come to this conclusion after years of observing the behavior and life styles of several of my truck-selling friends and acquaintances.

Take "Big Hearted" Harold, my main vehicle man. Harold is so happy all the time, always drives something red and brand new, and always is getting those little wall plaques that signify his prowess as a salesman.

Harold can demonstrate a truck and somehow convince you that it actually was assembled on a Wednesday with you in mind, and if you don't take possession of it immediately, you'll be committing a crime against nature, your ancestors and the stability of the nation. It is obvious that he enjoys his work, his loyal clientele and his nice commissions.

The truth is, trucks sell themselves. All the salesman has to do is present it properly to prospective buyers. Little things like parking the vehicle in a conspicious place, making sure it smells right and having the radio set on the proper country music station are all that's required.

The pickup boom will continue on into the 1990's and probably on into the 21st century, "Big Hearted" Harold tells me. Trucks are getting prettier and fancier every year, even to the point where lots of former BMW drivers now are cruising around in Chevy Silverados and Ford XLT Lariats.

We know that people are going to buy trucks. They can't do without them! Therefore, the only way a salesman can fail to sell them is to try not to.

"But you got to really know what you're doin' to be able to sell trucks!" Big Hearted Harold said just the other day.

Well, so what. You've got to know what you're doing even with the bad jobs today.

2. **Dermatologist:** His or her patients seldom get completely cured, unless they have something terrible and temporary, like poison ivy or chigger overload.

I am somewhat of an authority on the subject of dermatologists since I visit one a couple of times a year. When I arrive at his waiting room for my appointment, it is filled with other red-headed, fair-skinned individuals who are trying to undo years of sun damage to their ears, foreheads and forearms. Every visit he says the same thing.

"Your hide's looking better," he'll say, "but we need to freeze a few more of these garbage spots off your forehead and maybe smear on another month's worth of this special salve."

"You mean that $25 stuff?" I always say, visualizing that tiny expensive tube.

"Yeah! You still using your sunscreen lotion every day and wearing that big safari helmet?" he's scribbling constantly but touching skin only occasionally.

"Yes, Sir, I am."

"You lie! You're not putting that lotion on but once in a

while, and you're still wearing that silly feed store cap,'' he'll fuss.

It's obvious that he enjoys all this conversation and the nice fees he's receiving at the end of that five-minute consultation. Plus, he deals with such nice people. Everybody knows that redheads with freckles and fair skin are so enjoyable to work with. And they are patients for a very long time since they have the audacity to keep on going out into the sunlight and getting blistered.

3. **Bait shop proprietor:** Talk about a job with no stress!! The biggest worry he has is whether or not the crickets get sick and die. He also probably thinks about the lake going dry and if the animal welfare groups will instigate a bill of "fish rights."

I know of former big city, high roller types who gave up that fast-lane life, moved to the boondocks and opened up bait, tackle and beer shops on the lake. They don't make nearly as much money but they have a whole lot less to buy. Also, their health is better and they aren't always riled up and wanting to bite 20 penny nails in half.

When you deal with fishermen and hunters, you often are dealing with people who are on recreational trips, and their minds are on fun things, rather than trying to figure out how to beat somebody. Therefore, the atmosphere is one of frivolity and happiness.

There are a few key phrases that the potential bait shop owner should learn quickly, if he is to become a respected member of the group.

"Boy, you shoulda been here yesterday. They were taking fish out of this lake by the cooler fulls!''

Followed by . . .

"They ought to be really bitin' again . . . tomorrow!''

Also . . .

"Crappie big as saddle blankets!''

And . . .

"A feller from Atlanta caught one the other day so big it took two boys and a man to get it in the boat!''

This is one of those jobs where exaggeration is expected, but outright lying about fish size or numbers is respected. This will come easy for most sportsmen without any real practice.

4. **Consultant:** This is the age of specialization, I under-

stand, so we have consultants for everything. They are available for assistance in growing soybeans, keeping sewage lagoons working properly and for improving your looks. I even ran into a time management consultant one day while traveling up north. One of my clients accused me of being a consultant the other day.

"Why do you say that?" I had to ask.

"Well, you're hard to get a hold of, and, when I do get you to the farm, you tell me to do things you know I'm not gonna do, then you leave. Then, in a few days I get a big bill!" he said.

"Well, I'm no consultant, but if you'd get those cows out of the mud and then . . ."

"See! See! You're doin' it again!" he spouted. "You know I can't do anything about that mud!"

Veterinary consulting must be easy work, since the consultant does most of the easier work. But when there's a prolapsed uterus or breech birth at midnight, he is not available because he's not nearby.

My consultant friends make good money, or so they say, and they never have to rope wild, lame cows in the woods. They can schedule their appointments to their own convenience so they can take the grandkids to the baseball game or drive up to Grandma's place for a couple of days.

I'm thinking of trying this consulting business, if I can figure out something I can consult about.

5. **Large animal veterinarian:** Like any other job, this is a good one if you like working with livestock and livestock owners. If you don't, it would be drudgery. It could be a great job if a few things could be corrected.

If farmers were paid what their products are actually worth, they'd have more disposable income which would allow them to be able to spend more on better health care of their animals.

Better restraint facilities on farms in general would make my job easier and safer. It is true; there are more corrals and squeeze chutes than there used to be.

I am very proud to be a large animal veterinarian and I think it has to be included in the top five jobs.

31

The turkey almost had me for Christmas

I DOUBT if all large animal veterinarians have been as fortunate as I have been. My clients always seem to be putting nice things into my truck while I am working in the barn or out in the corral. I've found sacks of potatoes, sweet corn and a variety of other vegetables stowed away in various compartments in my practice vehicle, put there by some sharing farmer. But the most memorable offering just has to be the Christmas Turkey of '62. Tony Bertrand, dairyman, part-time pulpwood hauler and jack of all trades, was one of my favorite clients and best friends. He didn't like doing any of his own veterinary work, so I spent a good bit of time on his farm taking care of routine, as well as emergency veterinary matters.

If I was there for an early-morning milk fever or calf delivery, Tony's wife, Mildred, would make sure that I ate breakfast at her kitchen table before leaving. If it was noontime, Mildred would insist that I take nourishment with them.

Along about September, I noticed that they had a few young turkeys milling around the barn. Actually, they were milling around wherever they desired. I asked Tony about them.

"Well, those are for Christmas," he said, grinning. "That big one over there is yours. I was just gonna clean it and put it in your truck a day or so before Christmas and your wife can fix it for you and all your crowd."

"Why, how nice, Tony," I allowed. "We sure can use it. I know Jan really will be tickled to get a big, old bird ready for the oven."

As I passed by and made occasional calls to the Bertrand farm over the next couple of months, I noticed the turkey program progressing. The one that Tony had identified as mine really was getting fat. I was getting ready for the taste of fresh turkey.

One evening, a few nights before Christmas, Tony called the house about a cow that was down with milk fever.

"I got your turkey ready, Doc, so why don't you just pick it up while you're up here tonight," he suggested. "Tell Miss Janice to get the roastin' pot ready for the biggest bird she's ever seen!"

It was an especially dark night, so I drove right up to the sick cow in order to use the truck headlights. While I was "jugging" the cow with calcium, Tony was doing some late chores in the barn. A little later I heard him moving something around in my truck and then the door to the rear compartment slammed shut.

"He's in a box in there, Doc," he said. "Be sure you keep 'im cool now."

When I finished, Tony and I exchanged Christmas greetings and I headed home.

"It sure is great to live and work in a place like this," I thought to myself, "and have all these nice people for clients. They sure do take good care of their vet!"

When I pulled up to the back door of our house, I realized that the back porch light bulb had burned out. Nevertheless, I turned out my truck lights and headed toward the back door. It was darker than I thought.

About halfway to the door, I remembered the turkey that Tony had put in the truck. So, back I went, stumbling over shrubs and stepping stones until I bumped into the vehicle. I felt along until I reached the back compartment handle and opened it up. Inside, I could feel a large box that I moved with some difficulty, so I decided to open the top and take the cold turkey out for easier carrying.

The thing was alive . . .

At that instant, the contents of the box erupted into sudden chaos. The thing was alive! Initially, the massive flopping wings, gale-like bursts of wind, clawing feet and flying feathers scared me half to death. I recovered from the shock quickly, however, and started frantically grabbing for legs, wings, neck, wattles or any other available extremity. As my left hand and arm tried desperately to stuff and hold the wild fowl inside the shaking box, my right hand finally encircled his long neck. At the same time, a massive claw engaged itself in my right forearm and a long ripping, stinging and burning sensation traveled down to my wrist. I knew that my arm was maimed; I just hoped that it wasn't mangled beyond repair.

The turkey was coming out of the box, in spite of my efforts to convince it otherwise. The animal was as large and twice as strong as a 30-pound feeder pig! With that size, there only was one thing I could do. I grabbed the neck and head with both of my hands and started to swing the bird round and round like a hammer thrower in the olympics.

The turkey still was squawking and flopping wildly while I continued to sling in panic. The neighborhood dogs were beginning to react to the strange noise by barking, straining at their chains and jumping at their confining fences.

"What's going on out here?" Jan asked tersely as she arrived at the back door. "Are you all right? Say something!"

"Go back inside, I've got my hands full!" I yelled rudely, as I continued my bout with the bird.

The sleepy neighborhood was coming to life now, due to all the commotion. In addition to dogs barking, back porch lights were snapping on, and the inhabitants were appearing at back doors and on their porches, squinting their eyes to see into the darkness.

I had wrung the beast's neck until I was blue-faced and almost exhausted. Mercifully, I felt the neck bones pop and I released my grip. Much more flopping around on the ground ensued, but eventually the fowl's carcass lay motionless on the pine straw of my backyard.

A trip into the house resulted in much verbal concern for my spurred forearm which was cleaned and painted with an iodine-looking solution. Presently, Jan was flitting around the kitchen producing large pots and pans, gallons of hot boiling water, and barking out orders on how to proceed further with a turkey plucking.

About an hour later, we were the proud owners of a very large, plucked, gutted and adequately cleaned bird ready for roasting. The only problem that we had was size and space. The gigantic, defeathered, holiday offering was much too large to fit into the small amount of available space in our refrigerator; nor could we squeeze the thing into our good-sized roaster. Finally, I took it down to the ice plant and stored it in a large dynamite box until Jan could make arrangements at the school lunchroom to cook it in their large oven.

We enjoyed the turkey and even shared much of it with our neighbors, especially for several straight days of it after Christmas. We also appreciated Tony's generosity, but I never did tell him that his turkey almost had me for Christmas rather than the other way around.

32

Dreams during a spring thunderstorm

WE WERE in the barn hall, just sitting there on bales of last year's coastal bermuda, waiting for the hard April shower to stop. We were only about half through with the calf vaccinating, castrating and implanting when the downpour had commenced.

Carney Sam Jenkins, great philosopher and gifted seer, occupied the entire bale to my left. He needed extra room when he sat because he usually brought out his razor sharp Sears Roebuck pocket knife and whittled while he rested. He was a wild and unpredictable whittler. His knife frequently slipped as he carved, often landing on the floor or occasionally in a nearby neighbor's thigh muscle. Also, he was an incautious tobacco chewer who drooled excessively and frequently spattered nearby companions when he expectorated. And he did expectorate frequently and voluminously!

I shared a bale with Possum Miller, a young farmer who spent too much time playing golf. If he wasn't playing, he was thinking about it. I occasionally played golf with him, but his temper was just too intense to suit me. He frequently threw clubs during fits of anger, sometimes losing them high up in bushy oak trees or deep in the kudzu-covered woods. Several small trees on the golf course had succumbed after being attacked by Possum and his bent-up golf clubs. He was good at working cattle, however, and often showed up to help when I did herd work in his area.

The owner of the herd, Mr. Jimmy Throckmorton, wasn't sitting. Instead, he was nervously pacing back and forth in front of the door, fretting and fuming over the time lost to the rain.

"I don't have time for this!" he bellowed. "I got hay on the ground, a funeral to go to, a pig to cook for that paper mill crowd. I just don't need this!''

Carney Sam stopped his whittling, leaned forth, then evacuated his oral cavity by sending forth a torrent of a vile-looking extract into a puddle of water just outside the open door.

"Aw, quit yo' trompin,' Squire," slobbered Carney. "Enjoy this nice rain that the Master has sent us. We need this shower!''

Mr. Jimmy was known by several nicknames. Squire, Counselor, Judge and Professor all were used when he was being addressed. The reason for all these titles was the fact that he knew some law. Some thought that he had been off to a big law school up in the northeast somewhere, while others suspected that he had taken some vague two-week correspondence course he saw advertised in the back of a comic book.

I called him Uncle Jimmy since he frequently was a behind-the-scenes advisor and supporter of various politicians and causes. No area resident entered any political race without first seeking the counsel of Uncle Jimmy.

The rain continued to assault the tin roof of the barn, interrupted only by occasional spine tingling claps of thunder. It appeared that we had worked the last calf of the day.

"What would you do if all of a sudden you had a million dollars?'' I said, staring into the rain.

"Man, I'd go out to California and play golf at all those fancy golf courses I see on TV," Possum allowed. "Then I'd fly across the water, rent me a car and play all those courses in Scotland.''

"Aw, Possum, you'd get killed over there," warned Jimmy. "They tell me that bunch over there all drive on the wrong side of the road.''

"Well, I'll just get me a chauffeur then," answered Possum. "I'd be over there a month or more.''

"Don't forget you'll have to come home in time to pick your corn and dig those sweet potatoes," I suggested.

"Oh yeah, that's right. But I'd get me a full-time hired man and, he'd do that. What would you do, Carney?''

"I reckon I'd get me a brand new, red pulpwood truck, rip off both doors, and hang a big Poulan bow chain saw from the back standard. Next, I'd take a club and dent up the hood a right smart, then go out in the woods and cut paperwood."

"You'd cut paperwood!" screamed Possum. "That's what you do now! That's the hardest work there is!"

"You don't understand," replied Carney Sam, after another profuse spit. "I'd cut wood when I wanted to and quit whenever I got good an' ready. Why it might take me a month or more to cut a cord! Wouldn't that be a fine way to live?"

"What about you, Judge?"

"I'd build me the finest catchpen, with a roof, lights and a cold drink machine," announced Jimmy. "Then I'd get shed of these piney woods, line back cows and get a hold of some fine purebred Black Anguish stock from out west."

"Black Angus," I interrupted.

"O.K. whatever they are," he answered. "Then I'd build me a fine home up on that ridge yonder. I'd sit out on the porch and watch 'em graze and make money. Then I'd run for the state legislature."

"Doc, what'd you do?"

"What're you askin' him for?" sneered Carney Sam. "He's already one of the richest men in Choctaw County. He rakes in a mess of money at that sale barn up there, he works on all them rich women's lap dogs and he vaccinates thousands of dogs for the rabies every summer. He's got a gold mine! That's why they opened up that other bank in town!"

"Well, I'd use that money to pay off debts," I dreamed. "Then if I had any left over I'd write a book about all the liars and crazy characters that I run into every day. 'Course I'd have to pay some outfit to publish it."

"Liars? Anybody we know?" asked Possum, "or are you talkin 'bout that south Marengo County crowd?"

"I reckon that people are pretty much the same everywhere you go," I replied.

"Hey, boys, it's slackin' up," said a suddenly happy Uncle Jimmy. "Let's finish up these calves so we can get on with our other work."

We did finish the calf work but not with the same enthusiasm as before the shower. Somehow the wild dreams of big money, trips to Scotland, the power of politics and new pulpwood trucks interfered with the work at hand.

There's a good lesson to be learned from dreaming too big. Sometimes, when you come back down to earth, it makes routine chores seem terribly stale and undistinguished, especially when the rain is falling and mud is four-buckle deep on your five-buckle overshoes.

33

"Aw, Doc, she DIED!"

JAN had called on the two-way and asked me to pick up some items at the store. That's why I was standing in front of the dairy section, trying to decide whether she wanted me to bring home a chunk of Cheddar, a slab of Swiss, or a gob of Gouda.

I never have enjoyed going shopping, especially at the supermarket in a small town. Jan's instructions often aren't very clear to me, yet are pretty specific as to brand, price or size. I just like to grab something off the shelf and get out.

Another reason I dislike shopping is that I often run into clients who want to discuss at length, the ailments of their pets or livestock. Sometimes it is quite embarrassing to be standing there conducting a question and answer session on dysentery while fidgeting in front of the delicatessen.

While pondering the great cheese decision, I heard the squeak of a shopping cart and the clomp of hard-heeled engineers' boots approaching the milk cooler. I could recognize the sound of those boots anywhere as those of Carney Sam Jenkins, homemade veterinarian and living legend of Puss Cuss Creek Hollow.

"Howdy, Doc," he loudly saluted, as he reached for a gallon of Borden's. "Miz Doc got 'chu shoppin', too?"

"Yeah, you know how it is. She's got her hands full with the kids," I replied. "By the way, how's your neighbor's cow?"

Too late, it dawned on me that he shouldn't have been buying milk, and that I should have kept my mouth shut about the cow. After all, she was the community milk cow, a black Jersey. I had treated her for mountain laurel poisoning a couple of days before.

"Aw, Doc, she **DIED**!!" he retorted, his voice echoing

129

throughout the store as if he were wired to the public address system. There was instant silence, except for the hum of the refrigerated coolers and the whine of the butcher's band saw as it whizzed through a chilled carcass.

"Yeah, she **DIED**, graveyard **DEAD**, not five minutes after you left," he restated. "I sure wish that you had treated her for the **HOLLERTAIL** like I wanted you to do! Now I gotta buy this here high-priced blue john milk!"

"This happens to me every time I come into this blame store," I thought to myself, as I looked around for an escape route. There was no way out.

Aunt Sissy Bailey was on down the way at the egg cooler, opening cartons and checking for cracked eggs. I sure didn't want to talk with her since her old dog had just died of kidney failure in the clinic. I couldn't go that way.

I could see other clients slowly making their way toward the dairy department, many of whom already were practicing the questions that they were going to ask their pet's doctor. Each time Carney Sam verbalized a loud "**DEAD**," however, they would stop momentarily in their tracks, with mouths open and head tilted, as if reconsidering their decision to confer with the killer doc.

"Maybe I can go out the back way here," I thought, as I looked at the narrow opening between the cottage cheese and ham departments. The instant I made a move in that direction, though, Theodore Miller, the part-time butcher, made a move to cut me off. He was wiping his greasy hands on a once white apron as he blocked my escape route.

"Doc, about that hoss of mine," he commenced, "she still ain't doing jus' right. I wonder . . ."

He was cut off in midsentence as a Higher Being apparently interceded on my behalf. The lights flickered once, then twice; then glorious darkness fell upon the huge store. Silence, except for a few startled miniscreams and carts bumping into canned goods, ensued.

"I got a light," I stated quickly, pulling penlight from coveralls pocket. "Which way is the fuse box?"

"Back in the back, Doc," offered Theodore. Actually, we called him "Taydo" — that's the southernese way of saying Theodore.

"Hot dog, I can escape out the back way," I mumbled, as

I abandoned my shopping cart by the chitterling and tripe cooler.

"Where's the rear door, Taydo?" I asked, as we bumped into and tripped over crates of strawberries and sacks of Vidalia onions. "I got to get back to the clinic pronto!"

"Straight on back, Doc."

"Here, you take this light, Taydo, I'll see you later," I replied when I saw daylight through the cracks.

"Yeah, Doc, you go ahead, I know you need to see about the lights in the clinic. But this old hoss, she . . ."

By then, I had jumped over the pile of boxes, was off the dock and was jogging around the building by the drug store towards my always ready and faithful truck.

"Whew! What a blessing!" I whispered, looking toward the heavens. "Somebody is looking out after me."

Driving off, I could barely make out the figures of shoppers stalled in their efforts as they all congregated in the front of the store. Apparently, they were being held hostage because the power outage had caused the front doors to cease functioning. I felt like a jerk for leaving the scene, but I didn't have time right then for hours of seminars on pet care and dog training.

"Did you forget the cheese, Honey?" my wife asked when I walked in the back door.

"Uh, naw, they were out."

"Out! What do you mean out? No store ever is out of cheese!" she replied. "I needed that for our supper!"

"Look, let's just bundle up the kids, and go down to the Dairy Queen. Terri called the clinic this morning and said she had stuffed bell peppers on the menu today."

Several minutes later, we made our entrance into the small restaurant. We exchanged greetings with Terri, who was one of the owners, and one table full of out-of-towners. It looked like our timing was good for a relaxing meal.

Presently, Terri was at tableside, taking our order in between short stories about her purebred Hungarian terrier type feist dog named "Tofu."

"Dr. John, I know you want the stuffed bell pepper and . . ." she said. "Oh, did I tell you that Tofu treed a possum in Loren and Geraldine's yard the other night? I was just petrified . . .! You want the collards or grits, Jan . . .? Then the next day, he came up with a rat! Two sweet milks and one ice tea, right? Do you recall offhand when his rabies shot is due, Dr. John?"

"Naw, I've forgotten. But I know I'm starved, Terri. Could you bring one of those milks on right away — and a pone of that cornbread?"

"O.K., but there's something else I want to get your advice on when I get back," she allowed as she pranced off.

I just looked at Jan and shrugged my shoulders. It seemed like we couldn't even relax and eat out without having to talk shop.

Several seconds later, I heard the front door open behind me and the sound of footsteps heading in our direction. Then, Jan smiled and spoke to someone occupying the booth behind me. An arm suddenly appeared over my left shoulder.

"Thanks for the use of your penlight, Doc. The power came back on about a minute after you left."

It was Theodore, the butcher, from the supermarket. Now he had moved from his booth and was trying to squeeze in beside my little Lisa and me.

"Doc, I need to talk to you about my old hoss. She just ain't plum right! Reckon what ails 'er?"

It is a great honor for a veterinarian to have clients and friends who trust your knowledge, ability and judgment regarding their animals. Sometimes though, it is nice to visit the cheese store and the Dairy Queen without hearing about a dog with indigestion or a dead cow!

34

The broken pinkie

I HAVE decided that I am just an injury-prone person. For many years, I rarely sustained injury until the day I jumped over a hoglot fence and messed up an ankle. Since then, it has been one thing after another.

Soon thereafter, a bull broke two of my ribs, a cow fractured a toe, and then the lower part of my spine was cracked when I slipped and fell on a slick substance in a maternity stall.

Just a few weeks ago, a large, long-eared bull named "Freight Train," that was incarcerated at the state penitentiary ranch, became incensed at what I was doing to him. With a mighty stomp, he smashed the back of my left hand into the 2 by 12 board guarding the bottom part of the squeeze chute. The only thing that saved my hand from being crushed beyond recognition was the massive accumulation of soft mud and manure on the soles of his feet.

The feeling in the hand returned in about two hours, accompanied by lots of swelling and discoloration. I really meant to get it looked at by a doctor, but we were busy, and I kept putting it off. It finally has healed with no adverse effects except for some ugly red scars at the stomp site.

My latest injury occurred last week when we were doing spring chutework at Fred's place.

"Fred, these wild Brahma cows are gonna kill us all!" I remember saying the first time we worked them, a couple of years ago. "Why don't you stick to regular cows?" I had just been kicked, stomped, butted and bit at.

"But, Doc," he countered, "Ain't they so cute with their long ears and droopy navels. And they bellow so funny."

"Yeah, they're cute and pretty and different," I agreed. "But look at what they've done to this catch pen and my feet!"

We had just finished vaccinating, deworming and dehorning a portion of them. The remainder of the group escaped by leaping over, plunging into and through the fences that were as old as fossils. The corral was wrecked.

Fred is one of my neighbors and also one of my best friends. His professoring job at the college takes up part of his time, but his 100-acre farm is his pride and joy. Most mornings before 8, or evenings after 5, he usually can be seen happily doing various chores in the barn lot. He may be painting the old barn, walking among the cows or cleaning off a fence row. In the past year, he has been mending and building a lot of fences. The catch pen has been rebuilt, with Powder River gates and higher fences.

We were dehorning a particularly rambunctious weaning-age heifer when it happened. The horn had been scooped out with a Barnes gouge, and I was clamping the artery when suddenly the calf rammed her head straight up, trapping my left little finger between the poll of her head and the top of the head gate.

Within minutes, the then-crooked digit was bruised badly and so tightly swollen that I couldn't bend it. It was smartin' a right smart, too!

A couple of days later, I noticed only a half dozen vehicles parked at the new doctor's place. I decided to take a chance, so I wheeled into a parking spot and carefully removed the tape that I had applied to the finger the day of the accident. A couple of minutes later, I presented myself to the receptionist.

"Oh, nice lady," I grimaced, holding the painful left finger cradled in my right palm. "Reckon you can take a picture of this finger for me?" I figured that if I acted real pitiful, I'd get looked at sooner.

Been here before?

"Have you been here before, Sir?" she asked in a very business-like manner while staring at my coveralls.

"No, Ma'am I haven't," I answered.

"Well, you need to fill out these forms."

"All these forms? It's a good thing I'm not bad sick!" I grinned. The stone-faced lady did not.

"But I'll be tickled to fill 'em out!" I told her.

Some minutes later, after conversing with several

nurses and techicians, a young doctor dressed in white appeared in the doorway of the small room to which I had been assigned. His clothes were so white they hurt my eyes. He was holding the radiograph of my finger in his hand.

"It's broken, just as you thought," he announced, while holding the film up to the light and pointing to a jagged bone fragment.

"How'd you say you did this?" he said, flicking at a miniscule spot on his shirt.

"Dehorning a calf," I repeated for the sixth time.

"Do what?" he gaped, slowly turning his gaze from the film to my finger.

"Yeah, I was trying to clamp off a bleeder, and . . ."

"Never mind, never mind," he allowed, reaching for the telephone. "I've got to get an orthopedic man to look at this thing pronto!" Now he was pushing telephone buttons with great vigor.

"Wait! I can't go now!"

"What do you mean? This bone may have to be pinned!" he allowed.

"Don't have time today. I have a bunch of calls and appointments this afternoon. Actually, I'm late for one right now," I said as I looked at my watch. "I'll get over there the next day or so."

"Oh, no, that won't do!" he stated emphatically. "I can't allow you to walk out of here with that digit in that condition!" Now he was standing in the door, trying to block my departure.

"Look, Doc, I gotta go," I replied. "But if it'll make you feel better, we'll just tape that finger onto my ring finger. Maybe that will keep it from flopping around until I can get to the specialist."

He hesitated for a few seconds, then sighed and reached for a roll of one-inch porous tape. Seconds later, with the finger taping completed, I walked out the door.

"You understand that I refuse to be responsible for this," he stated, as he followed me down the hall. "If you are going to be so bull-headed and not take my advice, then why don't you just go to a horse doctor?"

"Sir, **I AM** a horse doctor!" I announced. "And I am **called** a **VETERINARIAN.** I also know that a fracture of the proximal portion of the second phalanx of the fifth digit of the left hand is not life threatening. I appreciate your help, but I've got to go. Just send me a bill if I owe you anything.''

When I pulled out into the street seconds later, the spotless young doctor still was standing in the clinic doorway. His mouth was gaped open, and he had a strange look on his face. I wonder what he would have done if I had told him that I was going to deliver a breech-birthed, half-Brahman calf at Walter Kirkland's place?

35

Don't use that left hand for six weeks

THE pager hanging on the pocket of my coveralls beeped just as I drove away from the doctor's office.

"Doctor John," our office receptionist, Susie, recited, "Chollie Kirkland is on the phone. She says that her cow Prissie is in hard labor. Please come to her barn at once!"

Chollie Kirkland is an animal lover. All her animals are named and treated properly as members of the family. There's Deerface, Meathead, Jessie and Johnette just to mention a few of the bovines. The hogs are called Fred, Tennessee, Bertha and Bulldog. Rex, Tadpole and Crawfish are members of the canine corps. There's even a mouse at the barn called Range Cube, since that's his favorite snack.

Walter is Chollie's husband, and he was waiting for me in the middle of the gravel road beside the barn. His hands were on his hips in the typical arguing stance.

"Where in the world have you been, Doc?" he yelled. "You said you were gonna eat a quick bite before you got here! You must've been to dinner on the grounds!"

"Well, I went by to see the doctor about this . . ."

"Just how long does it take you to eat dinner?" he interrupted. "Old Prissie's in misery and Chollie's bad riled!"

"I told you not to breed that big Beefmaster bull to those little ole heifers." I argued. "But you won't listen!"

Walter and Chollie are two of my best friends who would give me their farm if I asked for it. I really believe they would! But arguing and insults are routine procedure whenever we get together, even though it is all just good-natured bantering.

"What's wrong with your hand?" a voice yelled from inside the barn.

It was Chollie, peeking out through a crack between the

vertical boards. She was inside a stall, probably soothing Prissie's feverish brow.

"Nothing. It's just sore as a risen 'cause it's broke all up," I answered. "But I can't even get time to go to the doctor. Got to be out here . . ."

"All I want you to do is to bring yourself in here and deliver this calf," Chollie interrupted, "then you can go on to the hospital." Chollie becomes very, very impatient when one of her beloved animals is approaching the birthing process.

I said nothing. Instead, I retrieved my bucket and other obstetrical paraphernalia from the vehicle, handed the heaviest stuff to Walter and headed into the barn. On the way, I dipped the bucket full of water from the old bathtub trough and touched it up with a little blue-colored Nolvasan. I like using blue wash water.

$10 extra . . .

"Doc always charges extry whenever he uses that blue washin'-up water," Bubba Jack Davis had complained recently. "You can just figger another $10 added on the bill whenever he foams up his water with a nickel's worth of that blue dip."

Prissie was down in the stall, laboring hard but with nothing to show for it except the tail of the fetus.

"Oh boy!" I said to myself, "it's a breech birth! I don't need this to correct with this sore finger." Chollie was kneeling beside the cow's head, murmuring encouragement and soothing words into her ear.

"Everything's gonna be all right, Prissie. Dr. John's here, sweet dumplin'. Just hang on a few minutes longer."

"DOC, PLEASE HURRY!" she suddenly yelled.

"Settle down, Chollie," I answered. "I've got to wash her up back here, you know!"

"She don't need a bath!" Chollie allowed.

Again, I said nothing, but continued my examination routine. I was wondering how I was going to straighten out a fetus that was trying to enter the world in reverse. Soon, I was prone on the cool, red Georgia clay, pushing and shoving the little creature around, trying to get the hind legs out straight.

It wasn't long before I had one leg flexed and heading

backwards in just the right position. I grabbed an OB chain, attached it to the foot and handed the other end to Walter, who was standing by with a pulling handle.

"OK, now pull, Walter!" I grunted.

Before I could move my left hand, Walter was impatiently jerking on the chain.

"**AAAGH! WAIT! WAIT! WAIT!**" I hollered. "My finger's hung in the blame chain!" Somehow my sore finger was caught between the chain and the pastern of the calf. Why is it that when you have something sore and hurting it always gets smashed again very soon?

After several seconds of finger holding, complaining, grimacing and grunting, I plunged back into the job with added determination, quickly adjusted the chain and, with Walter's help, extended the leg into the birth canal. It wasn't long before the other leg also was manipulated into proper position.

The calf jack was positioned quickly and the little calf then gently delivered by Walter's experienced calf jacking technique while I yelled orders. Only then did Chollie abandon Prissie. In a flash, her attention turned to the slick, very still newborn, and initiated her skillful total body massage with a burlap sack.

Unfortunately, many calves that are presented hind end first often are stillborn. There was no sign of movement in Prissie's calf which indicated to me that the little heifer probably was going to add to the mortality statistics.

While Chollie continued her brisk rubdown, I quickly injected a small dose of respiratory stimulant under the little patient's tongue. Then I went back to the exhausted Prissie, checked for a twin and possible injuries.

She's breathin' . . .

"Doc, she's breathin'!" yelled Walter. Immediately all eyes turned to the little patient, just in time to see her take another breath and slightly move one ear.

As I stood there, the calf seemed to gain strength with each passing second. Soon she was snorting and shaking her head like newborn calves are supposed to do. It always is rewarding to see a successful outcome from a frequently chaotic and difficult birthing process such as this one. By then, Prissie was up tending to her new offspring.

I realized then that my broken finger was throbbing fiercely. Now that the excitement in the stall had subsided, the pain seemed to be much more intense and constant.

"I gotta go see about this finger," I said, while washing up in the bucket. "Looks like everything's going to be fine here."

"Doc, thanks ever so much," allowed Chollie, never taking her eyes off the new arrival. "We really appreciate what you do to help us."

"Yeah, Doc, we want you and Jan to come down here for supper this weekend. I've got all these blue gills we need to fry up and eat." There's nothing like good neighbors!

Within a half hour, I was having my left hand radiographed at the orthopedic surgeon's place. It wasn't long before the doctor called me into his private office.

"I reckon your work with large animals makes broken bones just normal procedure, doesn't it?" he said while viewing the X-rays.

"No, not really," I replied. "I've been real lucky to have avoided that."

"Well, what do you call all this?" he asked, pointing at the X-ray.

"This little finger here has two breaks in it. A fresh one right here," he pointed out, "then another one in the next bone. Probably broke that one a week or 10 days ago. Then look over here at these metacarpal bones. Looks like you broke this hand a month or so ago, plus there's a callus here several years old."

"Well, I didn't know . . ."

"What's going on? Are you injury-prone or something?" asked the doctor.

"Uh, can you fix this finger or not?" I asked.

"I need to cut right across the top of this joint here and pin these fragments back together," he allowed, touching the digit for the first time. "But, if I do that, it's going to be stiff since that break goes clean through into the joint."

"What about just putting a cast on it?" I suggested.

"If I do that, it'll be stiff since I can't get good apposition."

"Shoot! Let's just put a little ole brace or something on it. I need that finger to work with. If I were younger, we'd pin it. But at my age . . ."

"But if I do that . . ."

And so the negotiations went. Finally, we jointly agreed to use a funny looking finger cradle equipped with a velcro-holding device. It was a nice little contraption since I could take it off quickly if necessary, then snap back on before my wife noticed.

My finger healed up well, although kind of stiff just like the doctor predicted. I appreciate his skill and knowledge which provided healing just as I appreciate the great humor he displayed as I walked out of his office that day.

"I don't want you using that left hand for anything for at least six weeks," he had said.

I'm convinced he was completely serious!

36

The red coat is a prized possession

It WAS the big end-of-the-year event for the Choctaw County Cattlemen's Association. There were several hundred ladies and gentlemen in attendance at the high school cafeteria, and they all were in good spirits. Cattle prices were up for a change, and the larger sale barn checks had put a smile on nearly every face.

Unfortunately, the prices that livestock owners receive for their animals often are at break-even levels or sometimes lower. Therefore, when a nice profit is realized, it is cause for an unusual degree of happiness, pride in the cattle-raising business and unbridled enthusiasm for the coming year. As the crowd slowly filed through the east door, I was pleasantly surprised at how many of them I recognized, even though it had been nearly 20 years since I had been their veterinarian. I also was amazed at the number of new faces, some of whom I recognized as sons and daughters of former clients.

Memories whirred through my brain like old movies. When J. T. Allen strode through the door, he grinned, winked and pointed a forefinger in my direction in pistol fashion. I immediately visualized the late night, after-the-salebarn cesarian on a heifer that I had done in an old vacant, dusty, chicken house at his place. I had been so tired, but somehow I got the job done, all by myself. Later, I had given him a lot of grief because he was at home sleeping in a warm bed while I struggled with the heifer.

There were the Mahaffeys, the owners of a large ranch over on the state line. I always enjoyed their spring roundup and the long days of working the calves with Clyde's crew. Most of all, though, I enjoyed Dorothy's plenteous, noontime cooking and their sincere hospitality.

There was Billy Tinsley, the auctioneer from the Livingston Stockyard. I remembered all the long, hot and dusty Thursday nights and early Friday mornings testing cows at his sale barn. I snickered to myself when I recalled the time that he and I almost came to blows over a cow that was a brucellosis reactor.

James and Dardanelle Clark were there, and I thought of the time James had fainted when he received his monthly statement from the clinic. I had treated his large herd of cows with a new, expensive dewormer while he was away from the farm on timber business. Unfortunately, I had not discussed the increased cost of the medication with him before I sent the bill. From then on, we talked about the fee before undertaking the work. He was too good a friend to lose over statement shock.

Mr. Lanier, who had been my biggest client, was there with Louise and their family. I thought about their beautiful farm, barns and fine herd of purebred Herefords and band of quarter horses. I knew how proud they were of their son, Johnny, a veterinarian and the current president of the association. He had built a veterinary clinic less than a mile from the main barn which made his calls to the farm much more convenient than it had been for me. In my head, I quickly figured that, in eight years, I had made at least 800 calls to that farm.

I was saddened by the absence of many of my friends. Some have passed away, some are in bad health, while still others have moved away or have sold out and moved to town.

Hauled steaks out . . .

Soon, the steaks were being hauled out of the kitchen by Mrs. Knapp's home economics class and the 4-H boys and girls. The Choctaw County crowd is famous for their huge, delicious steaks, and this night they were just perfect. The rare sirloin they brought to me was hanging over the top half of the plate.

After everyone had finished with their steaks and dessert, Johnny called the association to order, and the usual meeting protocol was followed. Bankers, politicians and other guests were recognized, a short business meeting was held, including a treasurer's report, and the banquet committee was thanked with a big round of applause.

I found myself feeling more nervous than usual about this speaking engagement. Perhaps it was because it was like coming back home after being away for such a long period of time and the fact that these people had supported my family with a nice income for several years.

Almost like being in a dream, I heard Johnny mention my name and give a brief introduction. Suddenly, I was standing there all alone, looking over the great smiling crowd and speaking like a robot. Before long though, I settled down and began to share some of the strange and perhaps amusing incidents that had occurred years earlier to certain people in the audience. Nearly an hour later, when I was really enjoying myself, Tiny Sample began to fidget which told me it was time to sit down. Just like that, the long-anticipated event was over.

Presently, Mr. Lanier was asking for the floor and as he came to the podium, I wondered what he had up his sleeve. I was surprised when he presented me with an honorary lifetime membership in the Cattlemen's Association and a beautiful red jacket.

The Alabama Cattlemen's Association is the largest such organization in the country, and I was very pleased to be honored in such a nice way. I've thought about the significance of this honor a great deal the past month. In my case, I have decided that I earned it because of an accumulation of deeds, several of which I have listed below:

1. The delivery of at least 1,000 calves, with at least 50 percent of those having been done at night, in the rain, while lying sprawled in the mud. Also, half had to be lassoed. Some 10 percent had been in labor for an extended period and required great perseverance and tolerance for bad odors.

2. The replacement of 500 prolapsed reproductive tracts, 50 percent of which were in cattle tainted with Brahman blood. At least 50 percent of those were so wild and mean that a potential prolapse replacer would have to stand in front of the beast and make faces in order to entice her into the chute, if available.

3. Have dehorned at least 10,000 head of cattle and/or goats.

4. Had at least one squeeze chute disengage from the truck and turn upside down in a kudzu covered ditch.

5. Been very diplomatic when called to treat a cow down with milk fever, after the poor beast already had been home-remedied to death's door. Knew how to answer questions on hollow tail, hollow horn, tight back, the Murrah and others not taught in school.

6. Been kicked and/or stomped at least 100 times by horses or cows. Broken bones are a plus.

7. Have written 10,000 health certificates, a few of which were incorrect and drew terse responses from state veterinarians.

8. Have been called out of church service and other meetings for emergencies or perceived emergencies, at least once a quarter.

9. Got the truck stuck in the mud or sand on calls at least 100 times, most of which were at night, in the rain and in inconvenient locations.

10. Supported livestock associations by regular attendance at meetings, committee work and selling all those raffle tickets.

Never before have I owned an item of clothing with the value of this red coat. It always will be my most prized possession.

37

Junior's my favorite mechanic

PEOPLE always are making declarations about what this country needs in order for mankind to be better served. Some say we need more doctors, fewer lawyers or fewer spineless politicians. Others say we are in need of less arrogant TV reporters and friendlier gas pumpers. I think we need more backyard, common sense auto mechanics.

I'm talking about individuals who don't need computers or fancy machines with screens to tell them what's wrong with your sick pickup truck. They just know!

There are times when I wish I had taken up working on cars as a vocation — when I have just taken a new vehicle back to the dealership for a problem, for example, and the mechanics are unable to correct that problem. Or worse yet, they create additional difficulties in the intricate under-the-hood mechanisms of modern day vehicles.

"There's no such thing any more as a shade tree mechanic," the man at the new car dealership was quoted as saying. "You can't take a school drop-out and make him into a mechanic these days. He's got to be a computer technician, too. Our mechanics always are going to school."

Those statements saddened and depressed me because I always have thought that good ole boy mechanics are part of the backbone of the U.S. If we lose them, I'm afraid we'll be worse off, especially when it comes to smooth-running cars and pickups.

"Reckon how he knows?" I asked Jan one day when Junior, my favorite mechanic, had quickly diagnosed a mysterious malady in our old, wornout station wagon.

"It's a broken housing down in the carburetor," he had said. Actually, his exact words were, "a busted housin' in the cobbrader."

146

He had raised the hood slowly while I tried to keep the old junk idling. He punched a little, tapped a few times, closed his eyes, and turned his head to the side so he could hear just right. Even when he told me what the problem was, his cigarette never left the corner of his mouth. Ashes fell on the radiator, but he never made a move to remove the cigarette that seemed to be glued to his lips.

Junior is my kind of auto doctor! In addition to his magical knack of "just knowing," his appearance is perfect. He wears dark blue pants and shirts, complete with battery acid holes and grease stains, with the name "JUNIOR" patched over the left shirt pocket. On the back it reads "JUNIOR'S GARAGE." He's never worn a tie, except when he was forced to on his wedding day.

Junior has been a chain smoker since he came home from the Korean War. I don't recall ever seeing him without a lit Lucky Strike hanging from his mouth. He never puffs or inhales, and he lights the next one from the one in his mouth just before his lips get scorched.

Gonna kill ya . . .

"Them ready rolls gonna kill you, Boy," Sinkin' Jenkins had said to him one day.

"Ain't no worse'n that garbage you got under yo' lip," he replied, referring to the dip of snuff Sinkin' had in his oral cavity. It was one of the few complete sentences I have ever heard him construct.

After he works on my truck, I find ashes everywhere on, in and around the vehicle. That's why Jan refuses to allow him to touch her car.

The reason I and many others put up with his crabbiness, slovenly appearance and excessive tobacco usage is his uncanny talent under the hood of a car. He is a genuine, certified "shade tree mechanic." This complimentary term is used to describe those rare vehicle repairmen who have the innate ability to repair most any engine-propelled machine but resist going to work in town at the Ford place. Instead, they set up their own shop under a big oak tree out behind the house and answer to no one.

Junior and I became acquainted one afternoon when I unfortunately broke down, but fortunately it happened right in front of his place.

147

"Something just popped under the hood and it quit," I told him.

"Chevy?" he asked.

"Yeah," I replied.

"Busted distributor cap," he said, never looking up from the water pump he was replacing. His hands looked like they had been buried in grease for a month.

"Busted" is his favorite word. Other favorite expressions are "tore up," "mommucked up," "boogered up," "heathens up at the parts house," "idiot drivers," and "just a piece o'junk." He has a direct way of cutting through the extraneous conversation and arriving immediately at the bottom line.

"Son, quit moaning," he says to anyone who comes into his shop complaining about minor inclement weather or pot holes in the road. "Be thankful you ain't in a foxhole in Korea." He never looks up from his work during these pronouncements.

He doesn't talk much about it, but apparently he was a sharpshooter infantryman during the war over there. That may be the reason he absolutely refuses to work on foreign cars.

"Don't bring them Tiyoaters or Moslems in this shop!" he tells people when they drive up in one of those makes.

Apprentice named Bubba . . .

Junior has an apprentice shade tree mechanic trainee with him now. The lad is a chicken catcher by trade which he does at night, but in the daytime he is trying to learn the trade with Junior. His name is Linwood, but all his friends call him Bubba.

Bubba is a right good kid, but he has a long way to go before he can shine Junior's shoes. He proved this the other day when one of my colleagues drove into the garage with his new Buick which was suffering from a minor ailment. Junior had gone to the parts house and left Bubba minding the shop. He raised the hood and stared in awe.

"I wished you'd looka here," he declared to my friend. "Did you realize they put this engine in here crossways! Gollleeeee!"

"Boy, you get away from my car!" screamed the shocked owner. "Don't you know that's the latest thing?"

148

"How come?" asked Bubba.

"So us suckers will have to go back to the dealer to get it boogered up, I guess," replied my friend.

The man may be right about the day of the shade tree mechanic being over. But I sure dread the day when I can't drive down to Junior's and let him just listen to my truck out under the oak tree and give me an accurate diagnosis. On the other hand, if Bubba is going to be Junior's replacement, I think going to the dealer will be my only alternative.

I think I'll get a group of Junior's clients together and see if we can get Bubba into veterinary school or medical school where he won't be able to do much damage. At least he won't be boogering up my new Ford pickup!

38

Buying flashlights will break you

CARNEY Sam Jenkins, the gifted seer, great philosopher and homemade veterinarian said it best one afternoon while store sitting.

"Mighty few vets get rich. Fewer than that get rich doing vet work," he allowed.

"Ain't that the truth!" I replied.

"Well, I've heard of lots of 'em who are wealthy," an apprentice sitter exclaimed.

"Sure, but they either married it, inherited it, got it dealing in real estate, or running dope," he explained.

"But this one we got here in this county charges enough to be rich," someone else suggested. All present nodded in agreement. Some even nodded "no" but meant "yeah," as they sternly glared at me with lips pursed and pocketbooks secured.

"Yeah, but he's just got too many expenses. You know, flashlights and stuff."

I've thought about that conversation often over the years, and how accurate it was. Sometimes, a person with a third grade education is a lot smarter than a college graduate. Especially in dirt road sense and barnyard savvy.

Take flashlights, for example. It would be interesting to run a survey among large animal veterinarians just to see how many flashlights they have purchased during their practice years. It would no doubt be in the hundreds. Add to this the cost of batteries and you have enough money to buy a condominium on Hilton Head. At the very least you could make the down payment.

There are three main reasons flashlights are a huge drain on the financial status of the practice. First, the flashlights just won't work right or very long under barn, woods, swamp or cow-tied-to-truck-bumper conditions.

The beam of light it produces never is pointing in the right direction or focused on the proper spot on the cow, so it winds up being placed in unsafe places where it inevitably rolls off and crashes into deep mud, a foot of straw, or rocks. If an accomplice holds the light, he invariably wanders the beam around gazing at the rooster in the rafters or seeking a possum in a tree. Either that or he faints at the sight of the blood and boogers up the lens.

Watching a probable fainter holding a flashlight is an interesting case. As he nears collapse, the light beam first slowly drops almost to the ground but then briskly whips upward, pointing skyward as his eyes roll back in his head and the faint actually comes on him. That is, if he maintains the usual death grip on the light which occurs about 90 percent of the time.

Second, losing a flashlight is like eating broth at 30,000 feet. It's a predetermined fact that airplane soup will sooner or later be delivered onto the shirt and/or tie of the diner. Usually it will be sooner. Flashlight loss is equally predictable.

Why flashlights are so easy to lose is debatable, but the primary reason is very elementary. They are lost because it's dark when they disappear. Therefore, when the light is extinguished and it is placed somewhere in the night, frequently it is forgotten. I know of several that have been placed somewhere on the exterior of my truck never to be seen or heard from again. Usually, by the time it is remembered, the vehicle is long gone and the light has fallen off in the deep mud or smashed on the blacktop into numerous useless pieces.

Leaving a light at a farmer's barn is like leaving meat in front of the dog house. Neither will be seen again.

"That's my flashlight!" I told a dairyman one night as he held a familiar looking light. "See right here, I even scratched my initials 'JM' on the side."

"Oh no, that stands for Jersey Manor," he allowed. What a liar! He had Guernseys!

I stole it back, though, when he went to fetch a bucket of water. Of course, I left it on top of the corral gate at the next farm I visited.

You can chain it, clamp it, magnetize it and threaten severe harm to anyone who loses your light, but it is inevitable that the vast majority of flashlights will be misplaced within a week of their initial use.

Third, even if the flashlight can be found and it miraculously emits visible light, you can be assured that it will suffer a power outage. They are bad about having a brown-out at the most critical time.

"Just two more sutures in this uterus and we'll be over the worst," I remember saying one midnight. "Shine your light right in here, Alphonso, and hold it real steady. This is critical."

Immediately the light commenced blinking and fading, like a critically ill neon sign. When Alphonso quickly whacked it twice on his open hand, I knew we were in a heap of trouble.

"Go t' house and get some of those batteries out of one of Alphonso III's toy cars!" Alphonso, Sr. told Alphonso, Jr.

I've tried all kinds of lighting methods. Various types of hand held ones, expensive penlights, even those that strap onto your thigh, head, wrist or waist have found their way into and out of my hands. I really thought I had selected a winner with the one that strapped to my head. But there were too many wires and cables that were attached to a battery which had to be carried somewhere else on your person. Also, trying to manipulate the light with proper head movements was difficult for me, especially when I would get sleepy and nod off.

A friend gave me an airplane landing light that we rigged up to the truck battery. The 100-foot cord with it was handy, but it kept running my battery down and I'd spend the remainder of the night trying to get it cranked.

People frequently discuss the great inventions of the last few years. Some say that the computer is the greatest boon to agriculture and society. Others say the semen tank, or the Thermos bottle or smooth-riding pickup trucks have made for a better life for those of us who are engaged in agriculture.

All those things are nice, but I believe the greatest inventions have been electric lights in old barns and financially stable farmers who can afford fancy lights for use when their veterinarian visits on a night call. Still, I'm mighty proud and happy when one of the kids gives me a new flashlight for Christmas.

39

A night to remember

It was approximately 11 p.m. when I finally straggled into the house. Jan was in the old blue rocking chair softly humming a lullaby to the baby in her arms, and slowly rocking to and fro. Paul, about 3 months old, was fighting sleep, as usual.

"Bobby Joe Henley called about an hour ago," she whispered. "One of his big Charolais cross cows is in labor. He said to just come by and pick him up at the house."

"O.K., I'll just get a quick bite and go on out there," I replied. "Anything else?"

"No, it's been real quiet. Your supper is in the oven," she said, quietly.

I reached down and kissed both of them in their hair and tiptoed into the kitchen, the sweet aroma of a recently shampooed baby's hair lingering pleasantly in my nostrils. Little ones and their mothers always smell so nice that time of night!

I grabbed two pork chops and a couple of pones of corn bread, wrapped them in a paper napkin and started back out the door.

"Be careful," Jan's lips read. I waved, pulled the door closed gently, got into the truck and headed towards Bobby Joe's place.

Bobby Joe lived in the small subdivision on the west side of town. However, his 30 brood cows were on the old, 300-acre, heavily wooded family farm about seven miles from his house. This created a problem for both of us, since he didn't check on his cows as often as he should have. More than once we had tended to obstetrical or medical problems on his stock that should have been taken care of days earlier.

In addition, he had no corral, just an old, semi-fallen

153

down barn. Every time he had a veterinary problem, a rodeo ensued, with two half-wild cowboys twirling nylon lariats while standing on a truck bumper or hanging dangerously out of the passenger side window.

"Bobby Joe," I had fumed at him, "You've just got to check on this herd every day. When these cows are having calves, you can't afford to let them go! And another thing — you've got to build a catchpen so that I don't kill myself out here some dark night tryin' to rope one of your old wild cows!"

"I know, Doc, but it's hard to get out here every day. You know, the young 'uns have got to be taken to ball practice, music lessons, and then I like to play a little golf after work every now and then. Then I hunt and fish a right smart, too." He didn't mention anything about fixing a catchpen.

Five minutes after leaving my driveway, I was turning into Bobby Joe's. I drove right into the carport until my two-way radio antenna banged on the eave. Presently, Bobby Joe appeared at the screen door, along with a set of diapered twins and a barking, tail wagging squirrel dog. The dog was the only one wearing a shirt. I wondered why those kids weren't asleep at that hour of the night, and why the dog was clothed.

"Hey, Doc, come on in!" yelled Bobby Joe. "Les' drink a cocoler 'fo' we go!"

"Naw, let's don't take time for that, Bobby Joe!" I pleaded. "Let's go get this over with. I'm wore plum out!"

"Well, let me get a shirt on and make one phone call," he yelled.

"Who could he be calling at nearly midnight?" I mumbled to myself. "Probably somebody about a hunting, fishing or golfing trip."

The twins maintained their posts at the screen door, staring at the stranger parked halfway in their carport. They were grimy-faced and filthy. The peanut butter and jelly sandwich they were smearing on their faces and sharing with the dog made them look even more dirty and sticky. I wondered what **their** hair smelled like.

Finally, he appeared at the door, pulling a golf shirt over his head. With a wave of his hand, he dispatched the twins back into the house, and hopped down the steps into the carport. Moments later we were on our way to the pasture.

"Tell me about it," I said.

"Well, Doc, when I was out there this afternoon deer hunting, I noticed her laying down over there where you killed that eight-pointer last year. She had her tail up and I could see her straining an' all."

"Did you get a rope on her or put her in the barn?" I don't know why I asked the question. I already knew the answer.

"Uh, naw, I didn't have no rope with me. Besides, she's just laying' there. She won't be no trouble to git a'holt of."

Some folks never learn! A calving cow that is down and supposedly unable to arise, somehow always manages to make a miraculous recovery when the kindly veterinarian's truck motors up. This rising recovery by the beast is immediately followed by a 50-mile-per-hour sprint toward the nearest thorny thicket or cypress swamp. This sets the scene for at least an hour's worth of cow chasing festivities.

"Bobby Joe, I swear!" I hollered. "Don't you remember what we got into out here last winter chasing that old lineback Shorthorn? Remember me trying to head her off with the truck and running into that stump? This truck was in the shop for two whole days."

"Yeah Doc, and I feel pretty bad about that. But this cow's just a plum pet. I guarantee . . ."

My temper was slowly getting the upper hand, but I was trying desperately to keep the impending explosion at bay. So for the next few miles, Bobby Joe and I argued in moderation about people who expect vets to rope cows in the woods at midnight and also expect it done for little or nothing. About a half mile from the pasture gate, the conversation ceased and icy silence permeated the cab.

Seconds later, I turned off the road at the wire gap. Bobby Joe, tight lipped, leaped from the truck, wrestled the infernal contraption away from the post, then half dragged and half slung it off to the side.

"Go to the left, Doc," he yelled. "I'll just hang on the back bumper."

I goosed the accelerator and wasted no time in negotiating the vehicle down the rough and holey logging road. Soon, three rusted strands of barbed wire loomed prominently in the beam of my headlights.

155

"Which way now, Bobby Joe?" I yelled out the window.

I received no answer, so I repeated the question. This time I heard a faint cry in distance from where we had just driven. Quickly, I detrucked and played the beam of my coon hunting light back down the trail. Out about 50 yards or so, I spotted a staggering, frazzled Bobby Joe, hobbling in my direction. As he came closer, I could see that his formerly clean golf shirt was now smeared with mud and grass stains, and that his pants were badly ripped over both knees.

"What happened?" I said. Of course, I knew what the answer was going to be.

"You tho'ed me off, Doc," whined Bobby Joe, "when you took off so fast back there."

"Are you O.K.?" I asked. "Did you hurt that leg?"

"Aw, I sprained that old knee again," he frowned, as he bent over and massaged the knee slowly and carefully.

After considerable moaning, rubbing, flexing of the knee, and several steps of walking practice, Bobby Joe announced that he was ready to continue efforts to locate our patient.

We turned right at the fence and slowly headed the truck down through the brushy trail, going left or right at various points according to Bobby Joe's directions. Finally we came to a small 10-foot-wide creek guarded by a high bank on the near side and honeysuckles and brambles on the far side.

"We'll have to wade across the creek, Doc. She's right over there on the other side."

We loaded ourselves with calf jack, rope, bucket and black bag, then slowly eased over the kudzued bank and into the water. As we waded across the knee-deep stream, I dipped up a bucket full to use for washing up the cow.

In order to get up the bank on the other side, we had to get down on all fours and crawl on our bellies over a well-used path and through a small opening in the vines. It was a trail that raccoons and other small wildlife used to get down to water.

Bobby Joe went first and was progressing satisfactorily in spite of issuing a series of "ouchs" and "ohs" as the briars and thorns jabbed and hooked him in the back through the thin shirt. I shoved the bucket of water and calf jack ahead of me and followed, snakelike, through the crawl space. In less than a minute, I emerged up on the bank, scratched from the briars and wet from the sloshing of the now half-empty bucket.

"She's right over here, Doc," allowed Bobby Joe, pointing the flashlight toward a large pine tree.

"Where?" I replied. "I don't see any cow!"

We quickly made our way to the spot where the cow had allegedly been waiting for us, but there was no sign.

"Well, she was right here less than six hours ago! I'm almost positive this is the spot!"

"Almost positive!" I ranted. "You mean you're not even sure she was here!"

"Well, I think . . ."

"That's your trouble Bobby Joe," I screamed, "you don't think! You expect me to come roaring out here in the middle of the night, after working like a slave all day, and tromp around in the woods trying to find a lost cow that you should have had haltered and ready!"

I looked at Bobby Joe, and then looked down at my appearance. Our clothes were torn, covered with dirt, mud and grass stains. My arms were bleeding from all the briar scatches and three-fourths of my body was wet from the encounter with the creek and the sloshing pail of water. At that moment, I again questioned whether I was in the right line of work. Perhaps it would have been better if I had selected an easier job — like working in a dynamite plant or cleaning out smokestacks.

I could have easily bitten a ten penny nail in half at that point. However, I started to help Bobby Joe search for our patient by rummaging through brushy thickets and pine tree tops left by pulpwood cutters. After about ten minutes of searching we had not seen hide nor hair of the animal, nor had we seen any of the remainder of the herd. It seemed that I had walked a mile or more.

"Bobby Joe," I hollered, "this is crazy! We'll never find her tonight. Let's go home"

There was no answer except the whine of the wind in the pines. As I stood not moving a muscle, I felt that cold chill in my spine. I yelled again, but heard no answer.

"Now I'm lost, and I'll be here until daylight!" I mumbled. "Why do I always get into these messes!"

I decided to sit down under a big pine tree and wait for a while in hopes that Bobby Joe would eventually come back that way. By then, I was so confused and disoriented I had no earthly idea which direction was east, west, north or south. Plus, it was cloudy and the fog was coming in.

"I wonder if those high-falutin' vets up in Wisconsin ever get into messes like I do?" I thought to myself. "At vet meetings they all say that their patients are always caught up in nice barns and waiting when they drive up. Then when I see pictures of 'em in those slick-covered farm magazines, they are always pretty and clean in their white coveralls, and both vet and farmer are always smiling at each other like everything is peaches and cream. I wish they would ride with me for just two days!"

By then I was in such a confused mental state I didn't know which way to go. Also, I was getting right concerned. Jan would be worried when I didn't return home after a couple of hours. She knew approximately how long it took for me to deliver a calf or to perform a cesarean.

Several minutes later, I heard the far-off roar of an eighteen-wheeler, as it made its late night run on the lonely highway. Immediately, I started in that direction. When I intersected the creek, I challenged the brushy bank with vigor, waded across just as before, and continued my beeline trek toward the highway, carrying my stainless steel bucket in one hand and calf jack over the other shoulder.

Some thirty minutes later, I found the highway right of way fence, climbed over, and gleefully ran up onto the black topped roadway surface. Even though I was stranded out in the middle of nowhere, I wasn't lost anymore!

My plan was to head west and hope that I would come upon the gap into Bobby Joe's pasture. I just hoped that I wasn't already on the opposite side of that entrance.

As I walked and worried, I heard the sound of a vehicle coming from town. When it came nearer, it began to slow down as if it were going to stop.

"John, why are you walking?" What's happened to your clothes?" It was Jan! Why was she out here, and why was she concerned about the condition of my attire?

"Where's Bobby Joe?" cried another voice from the

passenger seat. It was Emma Lou, Bobby Joe's big, muscular wife. "He's gone and got himself lost in the woods, hasn't he?" she snorted with contempt. No wonder he stayed away from home hunting most of the time.

I crawled into the back seat of the car amongst several children of the two families. Some were asleep in the back, but others, including Bobby Joe's twins, were wide awake. I noticed that the twins were still eating on a jelly sandwich. I wondered if it was the same one they had been sharing with the dog several hours ago.

While I humbly confessed to our predicament, we motored the half mile or so and turned in at the entrance.

"Go right, Jan," ordered Emma Lou, "We'll go up here to the old homeplace and ring that old dinner bell. I always do that when Bobby Joe's hunting out here in the woods and I need him for something. He'll be here in less than 30 minutes."

Shortly, she was pulling viciously on the chain and the bell was sending forth its loud penetrating message into the depths of the foggy night. Sleeping children bolted upright in terror from the sudden racket, but were quickly settled down by the two grownups in the auto.

"Now we'll just wait," announced Emma Lou, as she sat back down in the car. Small talk ensued, and someone started fiddling with the radio. Apparently, I dozed off, because the next thing I remember was Bobby Joe crawling into the car on the other side.

"Doc, you left your switch on in the truck and your battery's dead," he allowed. "When I couldn't find you I was going to drive the truck on up here and ring the bell. I figured you had gotten lost," he sneered.

"And you weren't?" I asked.

"Naw, I was just looking for the cow!"

"Did you find her!"

"Oh sure! She already had the calf, and they're both fine. While I was here, though, I thought I'd just check all the rest of them out. I've got a calf limping real bad, Doc, and I thought maybe we could go and try to catch him while you're here. He's just a pet . . ."

I don't recall the exact words I said at that point. However, I was quite loud. I said something to the effect that he was a thoughtless person who didn't deserve the privilege of owning livestock nor having friends. Also, as of that moment, he should find himself another veterinarian to harass, since I would not be available for consultation or calls to his farm any more. I had taken my last nightly dose of abuse from Bobby Joe!

We left the truck in the woods and headed home. I'd get my service station buddy to come out with me at daylight and get it going. Bobby Joe and I argued all the way to town, while our wives and children sat quietly, with lips pursed, in the front seat.

"Send me a bill if I owe you anything," sneered Bobby Joe, as he and the family exited the car some five minutes later.

"You'll get a bill all right," I countered, "but don't call me again!"

I sat quietly seething on the way home. Jan said nothing until we pulled into our carport.

"Honey, I hate to see you get this angry," she said softly. "It's not good for you. You might have a stroke!"

Bobby Joe refused to pay the $100 bill that I sent him. I said nothing and wrote no nasty notes on the statements. However, when he opened up a new TV store about six months later, I was there for the grand opening. After looking around and pricing all the merchandise, I selected a real nice 24-inch color set in a beautiful walnut cabinet. It retailed for about $500.

"Please deliver this one to my house," I told the clerk, "and tell Bobby Joe to send me a bill if I owe him anything!"

40

Improving banquet menus

I HOPE what I am about to say will not incense any of my conference-arranging friends to the point of making angry late-night phone calls. However, it is time someone discusses the matter, and I do feel obliged to do so.

It's those agricultural banquet menus! Somehow we need to do a better job of serving fitting victuals at these events. This doesn't mean that all food at all banquets and dinners is below minimum edible standards, but improvements are definitely necessary in some instances.

First, nobody should be required to consume green peas. They shouldn't even be rolled onto the plate! You know the ones I'm talking about. They're those little dried up, wrinkled and half-petrified worm capsule-looking things that also have the appearance of diseased chinaberries. You can't chew them because of possible damage to frail teeth and the sensitive mucous membranes of the oral cavity.

If a person had a notion to eat something the consistency of ball bearings, then he or she should truck on down to the auto parts house or perhaps sneak out back of the filling station and scoop up some loose ones lying there in the old grease. So let's stop this foolish practice of trying to get folks to eat those silly peas!

Now I don't mean to condemn all peas or beans, just those of the green English variety. Black-eyed ones, pinto and great northern beans or even butterbeans are excellent choices for fancy banquet use, as long as they are cooked done, along with a chunk of fatback or a ham hock.

Second, the vegetables should be cooked. I have noticed that when I banquet with my friends, colleagues and fellow bovine enthusiasts in the vast areas to the east, north and west of Bowling Green, they have a tendency to undercook things. The potatoes are kind of like raw apples, the broccoli is similar to sorghum and the green beans are mildly parched. 'Course they are right good, in an odd way, but I'm concerned because it's uncivilized to consume those vegetables in the raw state if they're on a nice hotel plate.

It's OK to go by the garden and grab a handful of radishes, turnips, corn or cauliflower and eat them raw if you are going out to check the dry cow pasture or to see if the sudan has come up.

Third, let's eliminate sauces of unknown origin and ingredients on food, especially meat. Nothing is worse than hiding a nice piece of red meat under a dipper full of liquified paraffin.

"Just rake it off, Doc, just rake it off," suggested a colleague the other night at a big city cafe, when I gazed in disbelief at a fine hunk of prime rib that was suffocating under an obscene quantity of runny blue goo.

But you can't rake it all off because the stuff works it's way into the crevices and between the fibers of the morsel. Defacement of prime rib may not be a cardinal sin, but it's mighty close to it.

In order to be fair, there are some things that go well with, or perhaps even need sauce. Things such as stewed goat, braised carp or maybe prunes. Also, gravy or something has to be sloshed on top of tasteless things such as rice, grits or tofu.

Remember though, gravy has a way of contaminating and staining ties, light colored shirts and other Sunday apparel being worn by the diner. A lot of infrequent tie wearers are right uncomfortable when wearing one and therefore, are trying to eat with one hand in an awkward and unfamiliar manner. This is when accidents occur. They are just trying too hard to be polite and mannerly. That's why ties, when worn rarely, should be polka dotted or contain lots of brown and rust colors.

My fourth concern is the drink offerings. It is important that milk be the principle beverage on the table, especially at dairy gatherings. Its presence should be conspicuous, and it should be easily available for pouring first as well as repeated glassfuls. The pitchers or containers should be attractive, and for the milk to be enjoyed to its fullest, it should be cold.

I have no problem with tea, coffee or other beverages being presented and consumed at a milk producer's dinner. However, not serving milk at such an occasion would be like having Pepsi at a Coca-Cola party.

While we're on the subject of milk, let's have butter and real cream readily available. If people prefer oleomargarine and coconut oil-saturated cream substitutes, let them ask for them instead of having to ask for the real things.

Fifth, since dessert is such a necessary and enjoyable conclusion to a good meal, I need to make a couple of comments.

When the lights are dimmed and you observe a fire on the pie cart, be concerned. Real he-man dessert ought not to be giving off three-foot-high blue flames.

There's a lot of things wrong about this. What if the drapes catch on fire or a long-haired, slow-witted waiter gets his locks too close to the flames? Nobody could enjoy their sweets while smelling burning hair and watching efforts to smother it with 50-dollar tablecloths.

The best bet for dessert is pie. Bring the pies, uncut, to the tables and let someone there do the cutting. Clean knives should accompany the pies so that cutters won't be tempted to go reaching for their dirty pocket knives. Also, pies piled high need special long-bladed knives to slice through the meringue without sticking fingers down into it.

It's difficult not to recommend ice cream for large sit-down crowds, and I have seen it served with some success. However, too often it is soft and runny by the time it reaches the palate of the diner.

Perhaps an innovative approach to the ice cream problem would be to bring frozen cartons of the delicacy to the tables just as folks are drenching their salads with dressing. This way the cream would be just about ready when the regular food has been eaten. Also, it would give ice cream fanatics the option of taking in their favorite dessert along with steak, potatoes and salad. They could even eat ice cream first and salad last.

Please, let's stick to good cuisine devoid of gravies, green peas, fire and oleomargarine.

What's wrong with eating ice cream first? I think it would be a nice deviation from the norm!

41

Claude

CLAUDE is one of my "main men." We've been friends for many years, and I have spent many hours working with his hogs and cows near the town of High Shoals. I also have annually removed dozens of roasting ears from his corn patch. He and his wife are always putting buckets of fresh vegetables into the back of my pickup truck, and occasionally I'll find a box of steaks on the front seat from a steer they have fed out.

He is like many of my clients. If you try to help them out, they will often respond by doing nice things for you. If it's a late night calf delivery, or a cow with a prolapsed uterus deep in the woods where trucks can't go, or an emergency health certificate, most of my clients seem to appreciate my efforts. A few don't seem to appreciate anything I do, but thankfully, those are in the minority.

Claude and I first became acquainted because of a pig problem. He and his neighbors were castrating pigs one day when the nicest shoat herniated. He quickly put the porker into a burlap sack and came rocketing to town at breakneck speed of 45 miles per hour.

As he came into town, he spied me standing with a group of citizens in front of the courthouse. We all had just paid our property taxes and were not in a good mood. He immediately pulled into a diagonal parking place, ran both front wheels upon the curb and blew the horn while we just stood there gape-mouthed and post-legged.

"Doc, you better come over here soon as you can," he announced while detrucking.

With that pronouncement and after seeing dried blood all over his hands and overalls, I sensed there might be a minor problem.

Immediately the group with which I had been conversing followed me to the back of the truck, where we quickly observed movement inside the burlap sack.

"What is it? What's in that sack?" asked someone.

"Is it a snake?" Everybody jumped back.

"Bet it's a mad dog." They jumped back further.

"It's a plum mess, that's what it is!" replied Claude.

The group was multiplying, since people from across the street at the bank and the dollar store had seen the goings-on and had curiously hot-footed it over to find out the cause of the commotion.

After waiting until we drew a good crowd, I quickly and professionally opened the sack and peered inside. It was a mess! The poor pig was lying in a nest of his own intestines. Trash, leaves, dirt and seed were sticking to the viscera like it had recently been dipped in glue.

"Whooo-weee!" I exclaimed. "Just look at this!"

The bystanders were gasping, women were slapping their bejeweled fingers to their mouths in shock and small children licking on free bank lollipops were trying to hide behind their parents' legs. Still, none knew what moving mystery was contained within the sack.

"Y'all want to see this?" I asked.

Only a couple of the men dared peek inside. Even then they inched up and very slowly peered over into the opened sack. Just as the second observer got within viewing range, the pig jumped and loudly grunted, like pigs do when they are alarmed or want to alarm an unwanted intruder.

"Oof Oof!" grunted the pig.

The two men jumped as if a bomb had exploded! They went reeling backwards, stepping on other observers' feet and legs. Purses and cold drink cans were being knocked to the ground, while still other curiosity seekers were dangerously running across the traffic to get to the scene of the excitement.

"Can you fix that shoat, Doc, or reckon I ought to just put 'im out of his misery?"

I was somewhat hesitant about replying quickly, regarding my ability to replace such a mass of mangled tissue within such a small, warm and breathing carcass. Before I could quit scratching my head and reply, a man in the crowd spontaneously testified on my behalf.

165

"Yessiree, that doctor can fix whatever it is that ails that dog!" exclaimed a rough-looking, leather-faced man.

"It's a hog, Ace," replied another bystander.

"Don't matter. He can fix it up, I tell you. Shoulda seen my dog he fixed. That ol' dog come runnin' out to meet me when I got home from crop dustin'. That dern propeller caught 'im halfway 'tween his eyes and his mouth. Near 'bout cut that cur's nose off! This vetran here stuck a straw up each nostril, and sewed that nose back on there, just pretty as you please. Why, that dog's normal as me or you, right this day!"

I remembered the dog. The owner was a crop duster pilot from a nearby town. We called him "Ace." It was rumored that he had been a terrific fighter pilot in the Pacific during the second World War. I enjoyed observing his crop dusting skills and the uncanny way he maneuvered over fence rows and light poles. Several times I had stopped on a dirt road and watched him as he flew, no more than ten feet off the soybean tops, heading directly toward my truck. I could even see his head leaning forward, the grin on his lips and the devilment in his goggled eyes. At the last moment I would buzz away from the spray that his wings dispensed and he would climb almost straight up. He'd be laughing like a kid.

"Well, this pig is a lot different from a dog," I countered. "But let's take him up to the clinic and give it a try."

About half the watchers scattered in a rush toward their trucks and cars, in order to race to the clinic to secure good observation posts.

Many people are fascinated by veterinary surgery. It's probably because surgery is considered mysterious, even magical, and they are real curious about what really goes on when scalpel meets flesh. And since few individuals are allowed in a sterile hospital operating theater, except as a paying patient, perhaps barnyard surgery satisfies their curiosity.

At the clinic the young pig was physically restrained and injected with a sedative. After the patient was lightly sleeping, the prolapsed viscera was gently washed with warm water and efforts commenced to replace it back through the opening through which it had been delivered. However, replacing swollen gut loops into their proper

166

position frequently defies logic. The intestines obviously come from inside, but the body seems to reject all efforts to get them back into their rightful position.

Such was the case with Claude's nice pig. However, after much grimacing, poking and considerable conversation from the on-the-fence observers, I was blessed with success. Next, a few sutures were placed in the enlarged hernial ring, drawn tight and then tied. The edges came together nicely, closing the ring securely. A few sutures were put into the skin incision and that was that.

"Now, he'll sleep several hours, Claude, so be sure and put him by himself in the cool," I advised.

"Is he gonna make it?" asked Claude.

"Of course he'll live," exclaimed Ace. "Doc'll guarantee it, won't you Doc?"

Now I try to be a good veterinarian and practice good surgical technique, but for some reason it aggravates me when someone wants me to guarantee a surgical or medical cure.

"No, Sir!" I allowed, purse lipped. "This is a live hog, not a waffle iron."

"But what's the difference?" asked a fence riding know-it-all.

"Tell you what I'll do," I said. "If you can get Dr. Paul or any of the M.D.'s over at the hospital to guarantee their work, then I'll do the same."

"Yeah, but that's folks," somebody said.

Now I was beginning to get riled. I wasn't throwing instruments, but they were rattling on the bottom of the metal tray, evidence of my increasing exasperation. I knew that arguing with that crowd was a losing battle, so I grabbed my paraphernalia and stomped into the clinic. That night Claude called.

"Doc, you 'member that pig you worked on today? You said he'd sleep a pretty good while, didn't you?"

"Oh no," I said to myself, "that dern shoat has died and now this guy wants a refund on that pittance I charged him."

"You telling me he's still asleep?" I asked.

"Oh no, he was running around in the back of the truck before I got home. He's out there in the hog lot right now with his nose in the feeder."

167

"That's good," I said, relieved. "I guess everything's all right then."

"Well, that's why I called," he answered sheepishly. "That hog actually belongs to my wife, and she wanted me to call and ask you something."

"Sure, what is it?"

"Uh, she wants to know if it'll be O.K. for him to have a piece of watermelon tonight," he said. He was speaking in an apologetic tone.

"Why of course," I allowed, trying not to laugh. "Just don't put any salt on it, and don't let him eat the rind. He might get sick at his tummy and bust out his stitches!"

"Right! No salt and no rind. Thanks, Doc!"

Some six months later Claude came by the clinic and left two packages of pork chops. They were fine, but had an odd flavor. Jan said they tasted like her favorite fruit — watermelon!

On another occasion, Claude called early one Saturday morning. He talked in his usual calm and collected manner, even before he got around to telling me about the crowd of sick cows he had over at the other farm.

"Doc, you better come on down here, soon as you can," he had said.

"What's going on?" I asked.

"Aw, that bunch of cows over there on the east place got out last night and broke into the corn crib," he replied. "They ate a bait o' that corn, I reckon, 'cause there's four dead 'uns and several more down and in a bad way."

"Four dead! More sick!" I yelled. "Hang up the phone and look for a cloud of dust!" I get excited, even if the owner doesn't, when there's more than one dead cow at a time.

On the way to the farm, I reviewed in my mind all the treatments for acute rumen overload acidosis. I could pass a stomach tube and pump in laxatives or do a rumen-otomy. The treatment of choice, one author wrote, was to pass a very large stomach tube, then use a garden hose to force a large quantity of cold water into the cow's rumen. The corn, water and other rumen contents then are siphoned out.

The only trouble with the garden hose treatment is that the rumen overload cases I see are always way out in the bulrushes somewhere. The nearest garden hose and water faucet are at least a half-mile away. The author didn't offer an alternative in that situation. It was obvious he had not treated any cows that had broken into corn cribs or whiskey stills hidden in the woods.

"I found two more dead in the woods," Claude announced when I drove through the wire gap. "That's six so far." He still wasn't nearly as excited as I thought he should have been.

"Get in and let's drive out and look at the sick ones," I suggested.

We spied one down by the edge of the pond and went bumping down the rough field to her. She was standing still as a statue, with her head straight out and her legs in a sawhorse stance. She was severely bloated on both sides.

When we arrived to within about 25 feet of the patient, I stopped, grabbed my lariat, stepped out of the truck and let fly with the loop. She started to fight when the loop tightened around her neck, then suddenly her eyes began blinking erratically and her body began jerking likewise. I slacked off the rope just as she fell over sideways, her legs stiff as posts.

I started jumping up and down with my knees on the chest of the poor motionless beast, but as is the usual case, it was not successful.

"Don't hurt your knees, Doc," allowed Claude, "because I believe she just passed through the Pearly Gates."

I reluctantly stopped the resuscitation efforts, took one last look and hopped into the truck.

"What happened?" asked Claude.

"Heart trouble," I answered, pointing the truck in the direction of another seriously ill patient.

Again I detrucked, roped the cow and looped the rope around the door handle. This cow was different from the other one, as she was fighting as well as bellowing. I was finally able to make a temporary halter out of the rope, which appeared to be more comfortable for her.

A few minutes later, I was easing a stomach tube down her throat. Everything was proceeding smoothly, I thought, until I felt her body commencing the familiar jerking syndrome that we had just experienced minutes ago. Her eyes were jumping in the same fashion as before, and as I watched in horror, she also collapsed in the same stiff legged manner as her late colleague.

This time I was too shocked to do anything other than step to the side and gape at the second sudden death in less than five minutes. I didn't even attempt useless life saving procedures.

When I looked up at Claude, he had already returned to his seat in the truck and was calmly perusing the previous day's funny paper.

"Doc, I believe we'd save time if I'd jus' go get my deer rifle and shoot 'em," he said. I detected a hint of serious sarcasm in his voice. But when I looked up, he was hidden behind the sports page.

He was right! Even before I had started veterinary school, Dr. Berry, our home town vet, had emphasized the importance of not making matters any worse.

"If they're sick, don't make 'em any sicker. Whatever you do, don't be responsible for their demise!" he had said.

We treated no more cows that day. Although two more cows died, they did so without any human interference.

One of the things that veterinarians must learn is that some of their patients are not going to survive, regardless of heroic treatments or hopeful prayers. And there are times when no treatment is the best approach, especially if it requires difficult handling of the animals. Claude's two cows that I caught proved to me that the "treat 'em with something" theory is not always right!

42

Here are some excuses for being late

I REALLY do like my profession and job, but I hope that someday I can retire from it and the constant concern about getting to the next farm within reasonable vicinity of the appointed time.

My clients have their own ways of acknowledging my tardiness or, in rare cases, an early arrival.

First, when I'm late, I'm in a big hurry. I usually buzz into the driveway, with a cloud of dust following closely. I try hard not to slide to a stop in front of the milk room, old corral or dilapidated barn. Old barns seem to have a way of collapsing when I am inside them or even nearby, so I drive carefully around them.

If the client is present, he will make a production of looking at his watch and making smirky faces, as in disgust over the late arrival. Usually this is followed by a negative head shake and a shoulder shrug that seems to signal an "oh well, late as usual," attitude.

Some of my older clients, in addition to the watch and gesturing routine, will look up at the sky as if to check the sun time with their watch's time.

My father is in this category. He can look at the sun and tell you the time of day within 10 minutes. Naturally, on cloudy days that won't work, so he just determines the time by watching the Greyhound buses moving north and south on Highway 31. On bright days, he can even tell if the bus is late by looking at the sun.

These types don't need watches, but they carry them anyway just for purposes of decoration. A loud ticking Westclox attached to a leather shoe string is adornment enough for weekdays if it is placed on the breast pocket of the overalls. On Sundays, a nicer watch with a gold or silver chain should be worn to preaching.

Occasionally, when I'm late arriving at a certain lazy client's place, he will make a big show of faking sleep on a hay bale right outside the barn. Just last week this occurred; plus the joker had gathered several spider webs and stretched them from his hat to the barn door. There he was, all sprawled out, trying to imitate Rip Van Winkle. A blast from my horn quickly brought him out of his flim-flam coma.

Another favorite verbal barb is canceling the call to the law. This is done just as I drive up and detruck.

"Maw!" the farmer will yell towards the back porch, "forget about that call to the police. He's here!" I set my jaw and stare right at his nose while pulling on my rubber boots.

"Doc, thought maybe you'd had a bad wreck or got lost!" he'll say, real concerned like. What can I say? Well, usually I think of something derogatory.

"Did you come up here by way of them state line road-houses?" he'll continue.

My reaction to this type of verbalization depends upon the identity of the perpetrator. Sometimes I say nothing, while other times I'll play along with the silly game. It's easy to find a large dented-in place on the truck somewhere and go into great detail about how some drunk smashed into it just minutes ago.

On rare occasions, when I arrive at an appointment early, a strange reaction takes place. First, when the livestock owner initially spots my truck, he will stop dead in his tracks, with both mouth and eyes gaped open as wide as possible. After several seconds of this shock-like behavior, he quickly looks at his watch, or the sun, as would be the case with some I know. Then he shakes the watch, holds it up to an ear, looks at it again in disbelief, then stares back in my direction.

"This blame watch has stopped again!" seems to be the message he is trying to emit. "I know that it is impossible for this veterinary to be early for an appointment."

"This must be a miracle!" he says, just as I drive up.

What can a feller do?

I will admit that being late is one of my problems. But it is really hard for me to leave a farm while a farmer is telling me all about his cows or the operation of the farm.

Just last week, Walter H. called about a sick cow. It was a busy day, but I squeezed him in between two scheduled herd-work appointments. He had the cow penned, so treatment didn't take long. However, I made the mistake of inquiring about the cow's bloodlines, and so he presented a seminar outlining all the outstanding features of each of her ancestors, almost all the way back to when the cows had claws and grazed with dinosaurs.

I kept inching toward the truck, but Walter kept pulling record books from strange hiding places all over his overalls. I cranked the truck, put it in drive, adjusted the radio, and started driving away slowly. Walter's slow walk now became a trot, as he extolled the virtues of Angus cows and why all other beef breeds should be loaded onto barges and sent back to England, France and India.

"Late for a funeral!" I finally yelled, leaving him in a cloud of dust. He was still clutching record books in his hands like playing cards, and his lips were moving. If I had been retired, I'd have just stayed there and talked pedigrees with him until dinner time.

Coffee and pie or cold milk and Gail Daniel's famous Revel bars have made me late on several occasions. "O.K., just one more bar," I tell myself, "and one more glass of milk."

But somehow, that "one more" becomes "several" more, and that runs into the next appointment. There again, if I were retired, I could graze slower and enjoy those treats even more.

In the meantime, I will continue to make excuses for being late, some of which I think are very good. At this time, I'd like to pass some of these along to my veterinary colleagues who are afflicted with chronic tardiness.

1. "I stopped at the store to get a dollars worth of cheese and crackers for lunch, but I got into a checker game with Carney Sam Jenkins."

This works good for some clients, not so good for others.

I know a veterinarian who started out early one morning on an emergency calf delivery but didn't arrive at the farm until a day and a half later. He actually claimed he got caught up in a marathon checker game. I've never been that late.

2. "The telephone caught me as I was walking out the

door. It was the state veterinarian all hot and riled up because I got some blood and a little cow manure on those brucellosis test charts.''

Will somebody please tell me how to palpate, TB test, draw blood and perform eye surgery without getting just a little extraneous material on the paper work!

3. ''Sorry I'm late, but Loretta and Conway were singing a duet on the radio. It was just so pretty and all, my eyes kinda glazed over and I ran off the road into a kudzu patch. Took me awhile to dig out and unwind those vines off my tires.''

This excuse works well for those clients who are country music fans but not so well for those who prefer the opera.

4. ''That big ole state trooper stopped me again! And I thought he'd never turn me loose! I tell you, that feller's a menace to law abiding citizens!''

This is a good one if you don't use it too frequently. Also, be prepared to show the farmer a warning citation in case he asks to see it.

5. ''I had to run through town and visit my little grand-daughter for a few minutes.''

I have found this reason works 100 percent of the time, especially after you show them her picture. Unfortunately, this is an excuse only a lucky few can utilize.

I suppose it would be a lot easier to just try harder to be on time than to always be trying to find excuses.

43

Good people are everywhere

I'VE enjoyed this trip, Tom. How about you?" I said to
Dr. McDaniel. We were comfortably buzzing through the
beautiful North Carolina countryside on our way back to
Georgia. We had presented a continuing education
seminar earlier that day to a group of large animal
veterinarians in Raleigh.

"And we got paid!" I added. "That will come in handy.
What are you gonna do with your check?"

"Just put it in the bank," he replied. "How about you?
Bet you'll put it in your van trading fund."

"No, this van is in great shape, one of the best I've ever
owned. I haven't had the first problem with it. You know I
had it serviced at the dealership last week in preparation
for this trip, and they went on about what great shape it
was in."

"It sure does ride good," Tom commented. "Let me
drive for awhile."

I pulled off the state highway, we traded places and were
quickly back on the road. I was relieved to just sit back and
relax since the late afternoon sun was burning out right
over the horizon, making our westbound journey more difficult.

Just as I sank down in the passenger seat, I detected a
different sound from the engine. We were going up a small
hill, and it seemed the engine was making too much noise.
Also, we were slowing down.

"Oh, oh," Tom said, just as I sat upright and looked out.
"Something's amiss here, I'm losing power." He was peering at all the dials in the dash, pumping the accelerator
and looking at me for suggestions.

The van's forward progress became slower and slower
until we finally came to a complete stop at a country road

turnout.

"You smell that? That's transmission fluid," allowed Tom. "The transmission's boogered up."

"But it can't be!" I replied, repeating one of Jan's famous expressions. "I just had it checked at the dealership last week!"

Having vehicle trouble in a strange land is a very stressful situation, as people who have encountered this problem are aware. It's funny how many different bad case scenarios quickly run through the minds of recent victims of transmission malfunction.

I always have visions of shyster wrecker operators, fly-by-night mechanics and fake parts sellers, all aided by the local good ol' boy law enforcement agent. Of course, the end result is a half fixed product that costs megabucks. When I complain, a fracas ensues and I wind up in jail a long way from home. They take all my possessions, including the farm for payment, and I wind up a penniless bum.

"Aw man, what're we gonna do? Out in the middle of nowhere, right at night, and we've got to be at work tomorrow," I moaned.

"Well, we just came through a small town about 10 miles back. Let's allow the transmission to cool down for a few minutes, then turn around and see if we can get back there," suggested level-headed Tom.

After a few minutes of cooling down, the van did seem to take on new life, so we reversed our direction and headed toward town. However, less than a mile and a half and a long hill later, we again were stalled, this time for good.

"There's a farmhouse back about half a mile. Let's walk there and get help," Tom suggested.

"Yeah, I remember seeing a man and woman sitting out in the yard."

Shuffling down the long grade, traffic was sparse, only an occasional car or truck passing by, the occupants all staring at us with pity, or perhaps it was a long look of relief. Relief that the contraption dead on the roadside belonged to the nameless strangers and not to them.

As we neared the driveway, we saw the man arise from his chair and disappear inside the house, only to reappear less than a minute later. He grabbed two lawn chairs as he stepped off the porch, then opened them up and planted them firmly in the deep bermuda sod of the nicely manicured lawn.

"Howdy, boys," he yelled as we approached. "Have a chair."

"Well, thank you. We just . . ."

"Looks like y'all's transmission just petered out. I noticed you losin' power goin' up the hill there, and I told Mildred here that y'all'd be back in a few minutes. I went on in the house and called Joe, so he'll be here with his tow truck in a jiffy. Y'all want somethin' cold to drink? Mildred, go get these boys a pitcher of iced tea."

"Well, thank you, that's might neighborly of . . ."

"Where y'all boys from?"

"We're from Georgia," I replied as we finally remembered our manners and introduced ourselves.

"I'm Mack Williams, and this is my wife, Mildred."

"Pleased to meet you," acknowledged Mildred, as she arrived with a tray crowded with tea and brownies. "What kind of business are you in?"

"We're both veterinarians," Tom answered. "We've been in Raleigh to a meeting." I couldn't talk because my mouth was full of brownies.

"Vets? Yes sir, I know all the vets around here," he exclaimed. "I used to be an artificial breeding technician myself, so I was always running into 'em on farms. Why just last week I had one of 'em out here to tend to a cow. He was telling me about some of the funny situations he's always getting into."

"That's for sure," said Tom. "When vets, farmers and stock get together, crazy things sometimes happen."

"Listen, you two doctors, it's too bad y'all had car trouble, but I'm right glad you had it here. I need y'all to do something for me," Mack said. "I know you've both got on your Sunday suits and shoes and all, but I've got this cow out in the barn that needs to be cleaned off."

Tom and I looked at each other and grinned, but neither said a word for several seconds.

"Tom, I'd be glad to do it but I don't have a North Carolina license," I said. "I guess you'll have to."

"Yeah, I reckon it's the least we can do," Tom replied as he pulled off his red jacket. "Consider it partial payment for all the brownies that McCormack ate!''

"O.K., I'll watch for the wrecker," I suggested.

While standing there feeling a little guilty about Tom doing all the work, I heard the whining slowdown of truck tires on the road in front of the house.

"There's Joe now," allowed Mack. "Dr. John, why don't you go on with him and get your van hooked up to the wrecker. Dr. Tom and I will be on shortly."

Actually it wasn't a wrecker at all. It was one of those new type "wreck haulers," a flat bed that can be hydraulically lowered from the rear end, then the vehicle cabled up onto the bed.

Joe had two Sunday afternoon riding companions with him and considerable discussion occurred while they were peering down into the innards of my ailing van. It was obvious that all three were shade tree mechanics and proud of it. Each had seen vast numbers of other cars, trucks and vans with identical afflictions. The consensus was that the problem was the transmission, a fact that every Tom, Dick and Harry within a half mile already knew.

Since the cab of the wreck hauling truck was already full of three good ol' boys, Tom and I were forced to ride in the van, which was some six to ten feet higher off the ground than usual. It was odd and a little scary, riding down the road in an incapacitated and motionless van, looking down at the other vehicles that we were meeting. It was amusing to wave at oncoming cars and observe the shocked reaction of the passengers.

Joe had called his wife on the two way and asked her to phone the owner of the auto dealership. He suggested that we park the crippled vehicle right in front of door number three of the dealership and he would have his transmission man get right on it the first thing Monday morning.

Of course Tom and I knew nothing of this plan, so we were surprised when we turned off the highway into the big lot of the dealership. Minutes later, as we were unloading the van, the owner drove up in a new pickup truck, with a dog box in the back.

"I see you boys made it O.K.," he said. "Joe, when you've finished unloading, take 'em down yonder to the motel and check 'em in. I've arranged a room for them until we get this breakdown repaired."

Tom and I stared at each other in disbelief! Why was everyone being so nice to us? Was it a trick?

"Well uh, thank you very much," one of us replied.

"Don't worry now, I'll get Willie on this unit first thing in the morning. We may have you out of here by tomorrow night."

"We sure appreciate this," I allowed.

"Oh, no problem. We try to take care of our vets because they do so much for us. Besides, I got this bird dog in the back staggering and flopping around. Would you mind taking a quick look at him?" he asked, getting out of the truck and going around to the dog box.

"O.K. Doc," whispered Tom. "I cleaned the cow, now it's your turn to treat the dog!"

"Sure, be glad to!" I responded to the owner. What else could I say?

A quick examination revealed a large tick attached to the dog, just underneath the collar.

"Aha! Tick paralysis!" I exclaimed, removing the engorged arthropod and then putting it to sleep in an appropriate manner.

A few minutes later, with the dog gone and van unloaded, we headed out, this time with the good ol' boys in the back and Tom and I up front.

A couple of minutes later, Joe was escorting us into the motel and telling the elderly lady clerk to take good care of us. She was his aunt.

"Oh, y'all are the vets! she exclaimed. "Yes, I have a nice clean room for you!"

As we were filling out the registration forms, she was busy telling us about all her animals: cats, dogs, chickens and two parakeets.

"By the way, have you boys eaten supper," she inquired.

"No, Ma'am, we haven't," replied Tom.

"Well here, take my keys and drive over to the steak house. Ask for Beulah and tell her I said take good care of y'all," she said, handing over the keys to her 1978 Toyota.

"Why, that's mighty kind of you," Tom said.

"When you get back I'd like to get you to take a quick look at one of my parakeets. He hasn't felt well today," she complained. "I think he took the hepnoleptosis from one of the dogs."

As we squeezed into the Toyota and headed for the restaurant, Tom asked, "John, do you recall ever reading about hepnoleptosis in any of your textbooks?"

"Well, we used to see a lot of that in Choctaw County. It's a disease that looks kind of like hepatitis, but also a little like leptospirosis. So folks just called it hepnoleptosis," I explained. "You can't find it in the book though."

"Oh, yeah! That's sort of a first cousin of the murrah head and hollow tail!" We had a nice laugh about those strange diseases.

The restaurant people were very efficient, accommodating and friendly. Beulah's husband's second cousin, once removed, happened to be a veterinarian, so we were the recipients of an extra large steak and an extra portion of French fries. Finally with our appetites in hasty retreat, we walked out into the night and headed for the Toyota.

"I tell you, John, I think I could learn to like this town," Tom replied. "I've never seen folks so nice."

"But who's gonna vet that sick parakeet?" I asked. "I sure don't know as much about birds as you do," I said.

"Oh no you don't. You're not gonna sucker me into that!"

"Look," I said, almost whispering, "let's slip into the room. Maybe the nice lady will forget about her sick bird."

"Can't do that because we've got to return her car keys."

So we agreed that we had to examine the bird, regardless of our incompetence in avian medicine. But before going back to the lobby, we decided to stop by our room to call our wives and tell them about our vehicle problem.

As I was dialing the phone, there was a frantic knock on the door.

"Dr. Vet, Dr. Vet! Please open up! It's Junior!" a lady's voice cried and sobbed.

"What in the world?" exclaimed Tom as he rushed for the door.

It was the clerk lady, holding a dead parakeet in a Florsheim shoe box. She was crying and frantically looking at the bird, then at us.

"Oh, please help Junior!" she yelled. "He's not breathing!"

More crying ensued as Tom gently took the little

creature and laid it on the bed. Then he looked at me with that "it's-dead-what-do-I-do-now look?"

"Uh, let's give it mouth to mouth!" I yelled.

"Yeah that's right! Mouth to mouth!"

Artificial respiration efforts on a lifeless bird weighing only a few grams is impossible and ridiculous, but we tried. I know that we did our best in front of a growing audience, as the guests from nearby rooms began to congregate in the open doorway. Some were in pajamas, others in gowns and a couple of the women had their hair in curlers and their faces masked in strange creams or ointments. Finally, we gave up.

"I'm sorry, Ma'am," I'm sure one of us said, "but he's gone."

It's always unpleasant to inform the owner of an animal companion that the patient has died. Some people cannot accept the loss, others accept it more gracefully and are thankful for the pleasure that the pet gave. This lady was of the second type. Even though her heart was broken, she took the time to thank us for trying.

"Thanks to both of you for trying to revive Junior. I really appreciate your efforts," she said.

The crowd at the door was slowly dispersing, but they were shaking their heads in positive fashion, obviously pleased with our efforts. Of course, we were somewhat tense about the situation, but we were still impressed with the people and their manners.

Later on that evening Tom wondered how many more animals we would be required to examine before we got our van back.

"Maybe we just ought to open us up a practice here," he suggested.

The remainder of the evening and the next day was uneventful. I tried hard not to unduly pester the mechanic because I knew that the more time he spent jawing over the phone, the less time he'd have to work on the transmission. About 6 p.m. he called us.

"Doc, this is Willie. I'm finished with your transmission," he allowed. "If it's O.K., I'll come by and pick you up, and then you can drop me by my house on your way out."

"Sure, that'll be great," I allowed.

"I'll be by in about five minutes. By the way, when we

get to my place would you mind looking at my little girl's goat. It's been having fits lately."

"Of course, we'll be glad to. My partner is a goat fit specialist," I replied. Tom was grimacing and shaking his fist in my direction.

We did check on the goat and found that it was one of those Tennessee goats whose legs lock up when startled. Then they fall over in a spasm for a few seconds before they are able to go again. We recommended to Willie that he purchase more goats with similar medical curiosities, breed them and become rich selling them to weird people who want weird pets.

On our way home in the rejuvenated van, Tom and I marveled at the friendliness of the people that we had met the past 24 hours, and how they had trusted us with their animals and other property. We agreed that our spirits had been lifted in spite of the mechanical breakdown. It renewed our faith in people going out of their way to help others who are in trouble.

There are good people everywhere!